ROCKET®
YOGA

Your Guide to Progressive Ashtanga Vinyasa

David Kyle

Project Editor
Christine Fenerty

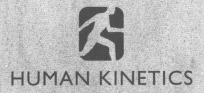

HUMAN KINETICS

Library of Congress Cataloging-in-Publication Data

Names: Kyle, David, 1980- author.
Title: Rocket yoga : your guide to progressive ashtanga vinyasa / David
    Kyle.
Description: First edition. | Champaign, IL : Human Kinetics, [2024] |
    Includes bibliographical references.
Identifiers: LCCN 2022052502 (print) | LCCN 2022052503 (ebook) | ISBN
    9781718216075 (paperback) | ISBN 9781718216082 (epub) | ISBN
    9781718216099 (pdf)
Subjects: LCSH: Aṣṭāṅga yoga. | BISAC: HEALTH & FITNESS / Yoga | SPORTS
    & RECREATION / Training
Classification: LCC RA781.68 .K85 2024 (print) | LCC RA781.68 (ebook) |
    DDC 615.8/24--dc23/eng/20221214
LC record available at https://lccn.loc.gov/2022052502
LC ebook record available at https://lccn.loc.gov/2022052503

ISBN: 978-1-7182-1607-5 (print)

This publication is written and published to provide accurate and authoritative information relevant to the subject matter presented. It is published and sold with the understanding that the author and publisher are not engaged in rendering legal, medical, or other professional services by reason of their authorship or publication of this work. If medical or other expert assistance is required, the services of a competent professional person should be sought.

The web addresses cited in this text were current as of September 2022, unless otherwise noted.

Senior Acquisitions Editor: Michelle Earle; **Developmental Editor:** Laura Pulliam; **Managing Editor:** Shawn Donnelly; **Copyeditor:** Annette Pierce; **Permissions Manager:** Laurel Mitchell; **Graphic Designer:** Dawn Sills; **Cover Designer:** Keri Evans; **Cover Design Specialist:** Susan Rothermel Allen; **Photograph (cover):** Weston Carls; **Photographs (interior):** © Human Kinetics/Weston Carls, unless otherwise noted; pages i, xx, 8, 11, 12, 13, 14, 15, 16, 18, 31, 251, 252, 256, and 263: Xinzheng/Moment/Getty Images; **Photo Asset Manager:** Laura Fitch; **Photo Production Specialist:** Amy M. Rose; **Photo Production Manager:** Jason Allen; **Senior Art Manager:** Kelly Hendren; **Illustrations:** © Human Kinetics, unless otherwise noted; **Printer:** Versa Press

We thank Veo Veo Estudio in San Juan, Puerto Rico, for providing the book's photo shoot location.

Human Kinetics books are available at special discounts for bulk purchase. Special editions or book excerpts can also be created to specification. For details, contact the Special Sales Manager at Human Kinetics.

Printed in the United States of America   10 9 8 7 6 5 4 3 2 1

The paper in this book is certified under a sustainable forestry program.

Human Kinetics	*United States and International*	*Canada*
1607 N. Market Street	**Website: US.HumanKinetics.com**	**Website: Canada.HumanKinetics.com**
Champaign, IL 61820	Email: info@hkusa.com	Email: info@hkcanada.com
USA	Phone: 1-800-747-4457	

E8815

I dedicate this book to you, the student. Inside, I hope that you find something to support your journey and that one day we may meet as we walk this path of self-discovery.

I also dedicate this book to my teacher, Larry Schultz.

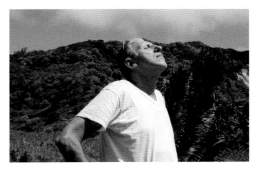

Larry Schultz
"Another day in paradise"
(1950-2011)

CONTENTS

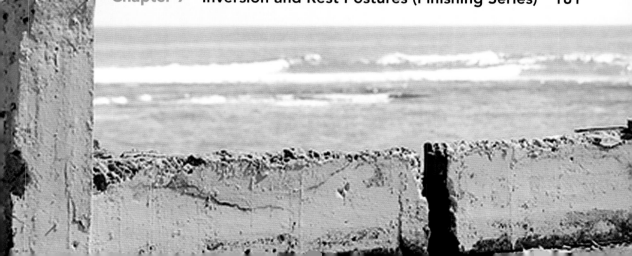

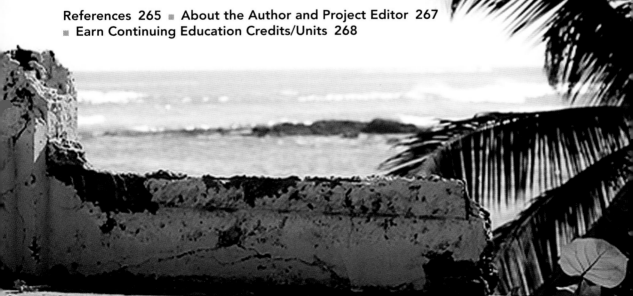

ASANA INDEX

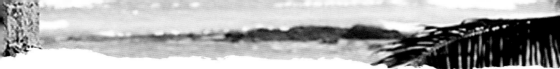

(continued)

(continued)

(continued)

(continued)

(continued)

(continued)

(continued)

(continued)

Chapter 7 Inversion and Rest Postures (Finishing Series)

Pose		Page
Salamba Sarvangasana (shoulder stand)		183
Halasana (plow pose)		184
Karnapidasana (ear-pressure pose or deaf man's pose)		185
Urdhva Padmasana (flying lotus pose)		186
Pindasana (embryo pose)		187
Matsyasana (fish pose)		188
Uttana Padasana (extended-foot pose)		189
Sirsasana (headstand)		190
Baddha Padmasana/Yoga Mudra (bound lotus pose [sacred seal])		192
Padmasana (full lotus)		193
Utpluthih (sprung-up pose)		194
Savasana (corpse pose)		195

ACKNOWLEDGMENTS

I would like to thank all those who have supported me along the way. My loving wife, Elizabeth Sallaberry, and my curious children, Lua, who shows me that it will all work out, and Dalai, who reminds me that it's not under my control. Without your continued support and love, I would have not had the drive to do what I do. You fuel my heart.

Thank you to my parents, Susan and James Kyle, for letting me explore things that were considered strange. To my brother, James, it's from you I learned reason and how to surf the edge without losing myself.

Thank you, Larry Schultz. Your guidance over the years refined me into what I am today as a yoga teacher, something I never wanted to be until you inspired me to jump on the bus. I worked many hours with you directly on this manual. It's time to release this practice to the masses!

To Reed Taylor, my first yoga teacher and the one who knew I was more than I thought I could be. Thank you for being real and connecting me with Larry.

Thank you, Katie Cariffe, for sharing your skill of detail and communication, which is essential in the facilitation of yoga and was the rock and foundation that steered the ship at 848 Folsom. Thank you to all the old-school It's Yoga staff and family: Maggie, Liliana Mieje, Chris Rosbach, Noname, Fred, Jimmy, Marlow, Tone. Thank you to studio owners who gave me a chance early like Maru and Otam who gave me so much energy! Pedro Luis, Yoshio Hama, and Mariangel Romero: Yoga is a union everlasting and free.

Thank you, Deb and Ian from Flow Yoga Center, for opening doors to the East Coast. Nina, thank you for opening the door to Spain and Europe. Leon London, you understood quicker than most and rode the wave. Thank you, Manuel Oria; you're the second in command of the mother ship in Puerto Rico. I wish I could name everyone I have practiced next to and been inspired by.

Thank you to Patrick Mccleaf for being a kind ear and being a friend who can sit for long hours throughout the night talking yoga, yoga, and more yoga like soldiers around a campfire. Thank you, Tiago, for being my fellow yoga pirate. We have scoured the seas and found the treasure that enriches all and not just ourselves. Thank you, Christy, Christiane, and Brandon, for sitting with me and supporting a mission to bring clarity and communication to our Rocket community. This book has helped our mission come to fruition.

Thank you to you, the reader, who is reading this right now—without your curiosity and dedication to the practice of yoga in the past, present, and future, the teachings of yoga would fade away. Pass it on.

I would lastly like to thank all our teachers who graciously offered to be models for us in this project. We are blessed to live in a time when we can come from all different corners of the world to contribute to the fruition of this book for all our students. We shared laughs and assisted each other in the difficult postures. In the end we only see perfection, but we know the grit and struggle that hides behind these clean images and the years of dedication and practice that each photo represents.

In no particular order: Manuel Oria , Ahmed Jabali-Nash, Christine Fenerty, Fabiola Maeztu, and Christiane Coste; I thank you from the bottom of my heart. *Jai*!

INTRODUCTION

To appreciate Rocket yoga and the progressive ashtanga vinyasa methodology, it is helpful to understand their origins. Ashtanga is a dynamic system of yoga created and popularized by Krishnamacharya and his student Pattabhi Jois during the early 20th century. Consisting of six specific sequences and practiced daily in order and under the close guidance of a teacher, the ashtanga practice was and continues to be a demanding physical practice.

Rigorous and exacting, classical ashtanga yoga develops discipline and awakens students' understanding of themselves physically, emotionally, and spiritually. However, many practitioners feel that the practice itself can be restrictive. Because the sequence must be followed completely, it limits creativity and honest expression, and it discounts the differences in physical capability and ability in each student. And because the student is taught each piece of the sequence only when the teacher sees fit, the teacher holds all authority.

Rocket yoga was born to destroy this false hierarchy and give power back to the teacher and student by urging them to listen to their inner wisdom to challenge and guide them in their practice. The goal of progressive ashtanga vinyasa further fills this gap with contemporary knowledge about the differences in individual anatomy and range of motion and with creativity, music, and freedom.

This book provides solid documentation of Rocket yoga—its history and philosophy, the sequences and practices unique to its tradition, and a guide to the postures and modifications. It includes tips for teachers developing their offering of the practice and outlines the basics of the practice for new students. Created to honor the fundamentals of the method as directed by Larry Schultz, a devoted student of Pattabhi Jois and the creator of the Rocket method, this book also serves as a standard of training for all students and teachers of Rocket yoga.

Contemporary vinyasa yoga is constantly evolving along with our understanding of the physical form, science-based research, and the needs of modern living. A blending of ancient wisdom with modern demands, this book is a road map that allows each student to experience and share the same sequences and philosophical ideas that thousands of self-devoted practitioners use to transform their experience of life through Rocket yoga.

Find a Teacher, Become a Teacher

There is no better way to deepen your personal practice than to practice with a certified Rocket yoga teacher. Rocket teachers have dedicated hundreds of hours to their own physical practice and understanding of the method and will be able to answer your questions and assist you in your asana practice. You can find certified Rocket yoga teachers at www.rocketvinyasa.com.

The website www.rocketyoga.com is the most thorough resource for the Rocket yoga method. There, you will find Rocket workshops and Rocket teacher trainings near you. Attending Rocket teacher trainings, workshops, or programs does not in itself provide certification to teach Rocket yoga or to use the name *Rocket*.

Only certified Rocket yoga teachers in good standing are permitted to use *Rocket yoga* to describe their yoga programs or classes. The term *in good standing* as employed by Progressive Ashtanga Vinyasa Yoga School (PAVYS) means that certified teachers

- teach in the method set forth by Larry Schultz without changing core methodology,
- maintain an active state in their association via directory membership,
- receive continuing education from PAVYS or from an intermediate or advanced Rocket teacher or teachers, and
- are mindful of the ethical guidelines laid out by PAVYS and have signed the certification mark and ethics agreement.

Only once they have passed the level I assessment are they considered a certified Rocket yoga teacher, and only at that point can they call their classes *Rocket yoga*. Teachers in training or teachers who use Rocket as an inspiration for their vinyasa classes may refer to their classes as *Rocket-inspired yoga*.

Whether you are looking for a teacher or seeking to become a teacher, the Rocket philosophy asks that we all remain students in our curiosity and our search for higher truths.

PART I

THE PROGRESSIVE ASHTANGA METHOD

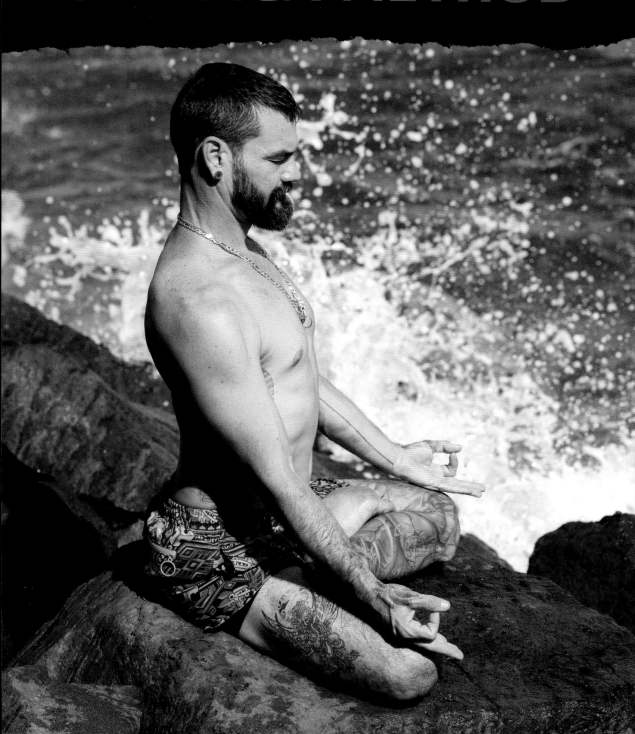

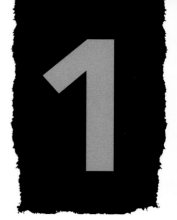

The History and Philosophy of Rocket Yoga

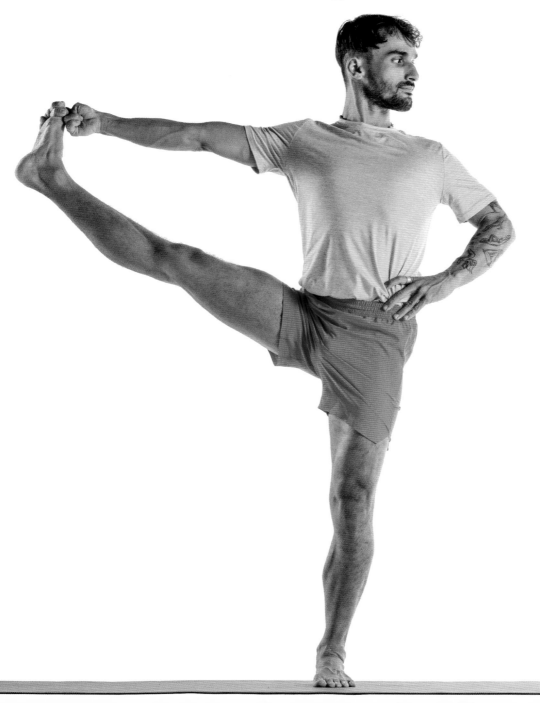

All forms of modern yoga can trace their lineage back to more ancient roots. Understanding the evolution of the practice provides a framework for appreciating the unique details that allow a particular method to resonate with us. Rocket yoga is no exception. From its roots in classical ashtanga to the creation of a new practice that celebrates self-expression, Rocket yoga as developed by Larry Schultz bridges the gap between traditional practices born in India and modern American culture. Progressive ashtanga yoga further brings together traditional practices and modern ideologies through the creation of a system that combines classical ashtanga and Rocket yoga to reap the benefits of both.

The History of Ashtanga Yoga

Ashtanga yoga refers to both the style of practicing a set sequence of postures as well as the eight-limbed spiritual path outlined by Patanjali, the ancient Indian sage who wrote the *Yoga Sutras*.

Tirumalai Krishnamacharya, an Indian ayurvedic healer and yoga teacher, is credited as the source of most of the yoga that is now taught in the West. Among his students were T.K.V. Desikachar, who taught a style of viniyoga that offered yoga as therapy; B.K.S. Iyengar, who established the alignment-focused Iyengar yoga; and Sri K. Pattabhi Jois, who founded ashtanga yoga as it is known today.

Jois' dedication to the teachings of Krishnamacharya and his diligence in preserving the tradition exactly as he had learned it is the foundation of today's ashtanga vinyasa yoga.

Ashtanga Yoga as a Physical Practice

Jois' ashtanga yoga is a dynamic and physically challenging form of hatha yoga that demands discipline. It is traditionally practiced six days a week, with time off for full moons and new moons and for women during their menstrual cycle. In the Mysore style, classical ashtanga is practiced under the guidance of a teacher. The teacher guides students through their practice by offering new poses in the sequences when they are ready for them and by helping with hands-on adjustments for each student. The physical practice of ashtanga yoga works to cleanse the body and mind, freeing them from not only physical maladies but also the six spiritual poisons: kama (desire), krodha (anger), moha (delusion), lobha (greed), matsarya (envy), and mada (sloth).

Today, it is possible to find ashtanga classes at many studios. These 60- to 75-minute classes are led by a teacher who guides the class through either the full primary series or a modified primary series. These sequences are composed of specific poses in the order set by Krishnamacharya and

Jois decades ago. These traditional set sequences form the backbone of much of the variations of vinyasa yoga today.

The Eight Limbs of Ashtanga Yoga

As a spiritual practice, ashtanga yoga literally translates to "the union of eight limbs." *Yoga Sutras*, Patanjali's classification of ashtanga yoga, outlines eight aspects that together bring peace of mind and stillness in the practitioner (see figure 1.1). The daily practice of asana is the gateway through which one can access the other limbs more readily. This is why nearly all styles of yoga begin with physical movement.

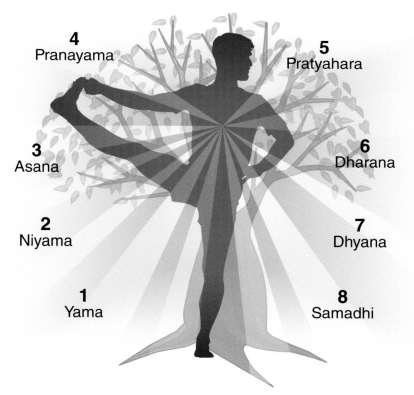

Figure 1.1   The eight limbs of ashtanga yoga.

Yama: Personal Observations

The first limb of living a yogic life is the observation of the yamas—the social restrictions and moral codes to live by. These concepts cover values for living a good life beyond what common law might require.

- *Ahimsa*—nonviolence, which includes physical violence toward others as well as toward yourself. This also extends to violent thoughts or ideas, self-harming behaviors, and how animals are treated.
- *Satya*—truthfulness in speech and with your dealings toward others in addition to living a life that is true to your purpose, following your values, and being honest in all relationships.
- *Asteya*—not stealing refers to the physical act of not taking something that does not belong to you as well as not taking credit for ideas or thoughts that are not your own.
- *Brahmacharya*—moderation in all things, whether it be in what you eat, how you live as part of a community, or the activities you partake in. This also extends to moderation in sexual activities.
- *Aparigraha*—translated as "nonattachment," this is the practice of nonpossessiveness and allowing others to be free agents and not subject to your control. It also means refraining from addictive behaviors that cause attachments or being stubborn in your beliefs to the point of extremism.

Niyama: Ethical Observations

Niyama is Sanskrit for "rules, guidelines, or observances." Together with the yamas, they form the philosophical basis for how to practice yoga in daily life.

- *Saucha*—cleanliness, both physical cleanliness of the body and your surroundings as well as cleanliness of thought.
- *Santosha*—translated as "contentment," this is the practice of gratitude, practicing nonjudgment, and seeking satisfaction in each moment.
- *Tapas*—a fiery physical cleansing through rigorous physical activity, this is the practice of self-discipline and willingly doing challenging things in order to strengthen the inner will.
- *Svadhyaya*—the practice of continual learning in a quest to better know yourself and your purpose in this life.
- *Ishvarapranidhana*—a devotion to a higher state of transformation, this means taking the time to connect to your higher power or your beliefs. If you don't believe in a religious spirituality, spending time in nature can also connect you to a power larger than yourself.

Asana: Postures and Bandhas

Postures and internal locks, known as bandhas, are used to create a balance in your body and prepare it for the storage of prana, or energy. Physical movement through asana releases blockages (granthis) that disrupt the flow of prana in your physical and subtle bodies (the energetics within the body), curing pain, disease, and other ailments. It is through the practice of asana that the other limbs become more attainable.

Pranayama: Energy Control Expansion

A breathing exercise creates a set intention of consciousness between the physical body and emotional mind. It clears thoughts and opens the door for higher realms of thought and deeper realms of ashtanga yoga. A breathing exercise also benefits health and general well-being. Dedicated practice develops endurance and gives the yogi ability to focus the mind and achieve a deep understanding of the self.

Pratyahara: Sense Control

The senses are used to understand the outside world. They can also be used to observe your inner world. You control distraction that arises from external stimuli and direct your senses internally to become more aware of what is closer to you than anything else—yourself.

Dharana: Concentration

Concentration follows this pattern: from the many to the few, from the few to the one, eventually to none. People have the tendency to think of many things at once. To concentrate is to pour all of your ability into one action. This action can be physical through movement or mental through a thought. Through direct attention with 100 percent of yourself, you can become aware of the object you perceive. In yoga asana, the body is the object being concentrated on.

Dhyana: Meditation

Let it all go: no mind, no perception. This is the state of stilling the mind. All perceptions, observations, intuitions, emotions, and anything that could be put into words disappear.

Samadhi: Liberation

Patanjali described many levels of this, some of which lead to the idea of liberation from certain obstacles. The ultimate form is liberation or freedom from all—to become one with the ultimate object of perception. Atman (God within) and Brahma (God in all) become united as one. Here this concept of God is open to interpretation, and some believe death itself is this liberation from life.

Tracing Your Lineage

Yogic knowledge, both physical and spiritual, is passed from teacher to student in an unbroken chain that links practitioners today with the ancient sages of the past. This lineage is referred to as *parampara*. My passion for the Rocket style of yoga and the progressive ashtanga yoga method is a result of my direct relationship and study with Larry Schultz and Schultz's direct relationship to Jois and so on, as you can see here:

1 Tirumalai Krishnamacharya
Mysore, India

An Indian scholar, ayurvedic healer, and yoga teacher, Krishnamacharya is considered by many to be the architect of modern vinyasa yoga, including ashtanga vinyasa. Born in 1888, he wrote four books on yoga, emphasized the importance of breath and linking it with yoga postures, and contributed to the revival of hatha yoga. Krishnamacharya continued to teach and heal until his death at the age of 100.

2 K. Pattabhi Jois
Mysore, India

Jois developed and popularized the flowing style of yoga known as *ashtanga vinyasa* through his shala in Mysore, India. In 1948, he established the Ashtanga Yoga Research Institute in Mysore and directly taught many of the modern yoga teachers.

3 Larry Schultz
San Francisco, California

After studying with K. Pattabhi Jois for many years, Larry Schultz returned to San Francisco and taught a style of yoga that he felt provided a more accessible practice to his students. While touring with the Grateful Dead as their personal yoga teacher, the term *Rocket yoga* was coined to refer to the style he developed and taught.

4 David Kyle
San Juan, Puerto Rico

For the past two decades, David Kyle has dedicated himself to the study and advancement of Rocket yoga. He established the Ashtanga Yoga Puerto Rico school, where he can be found daily practicing and teaching Rocket yoga as well as classical ashtanga yoga.

Tracing your own yogic lineage is a practice in humility that recognizes where your knowledge comes from and a source of pride that connects you to a continuing legacy. Using my lineage as a guide, outline your unique lineage back to Krishnamacharya. List only the teachers you feel truly affect and inspire your yoga journey. It may be useful to describe in a sentence or two what you have learned from that teacher.

The Birth of Rocket Yoga

The birth of Rocket yoga is the story of Larry Schultz's yoga journey, from his personal transformation through the practice of yoga to how he wanted to share his love of the practice with others. Schultz first encountered yoga while on vacation in the Caribbean when he was 29 years old. As he tells it, he glanced over to a rock where an older gentleman named Cliff was practicing yoga outside. "I ran over to him and said, 'Dude, what were you doing on that rock?'" Schultz said. "He said, 'Yoga, ashtanga yoga.' Out of the corner of my eye I saw he had a young girlfriend. I interpreted it in my head that you could be healthy in old age and have love in old age. Most people who are old don't have health and love late in life. [And that's what] Cliff demonstrated. And that's what I wanted" (Russel 2018). His curiosity ignited, Schultz returned to his hometown of Austin, Texas, and began diligently practicing yoga.

Schultz was intrigued by ashtanga yoga—the challenge of the physical practice and the connection to spirit. When Pattabhi Jois came to Austin in 1982 for an ashtanga workshop hosted by studio owner Stan Hafner, Schultz signed up. This meeting between Schultz and Jois ignited a yearslong study in which Schultz traveled to Mysore, India, multiple times to study directly with Jois and continued to attend workshops with him in the United States for many years.

In an article in *Yogi Times*, Schultz remembered an experience with Jois. "Pattabhi said there were three kinds of yoga students," Schultz remembers. "He told us, 'The first kind, all is coming in seven years; the second kind, all is coming in 12 years; and the third kind, bad people.' He looks at me and he says, '25 years, all is coming.' I said Oh f***! But I walked out and thought, well when I'm 56 my whole life is going to be completely different. And it is. It's remarkable" (Crooks 2017). It was always amusing to Schultz to reflect on where yoga first found him and where it took him in his life. From years of diligent practice under Jois, Schultz changed his habits. He cleaned up his lifestyle and felt a calling to share his life-changing experience with others. He decided that he would teach.

In 1989, Schultz began teaching ashtanga vinyasa yoga in San Francisco, becoming one of the first students of Jois to teach the system. He also became one of the first to open a yoga studio with the goal of making ashtanga yoga accessible to everyone, both physically and financially. And then he did what was unthinkable to the traditionalists—he began to revise the system itself.

Classical ashtanga was built on a hierarchy—not only of postures and series but of teachers as well. Schultz believed that the classical ashtanga system did not resonate with the needs of his students, and by breaking with the hierarchies of ashtanga tradition and allowing all students to have access to all poses, he could provide a system that capitalized on each person's strengths. This was in conflict with Jois' Mysore style, in which only authorized teachers were allowed to give a student a new pose to practice after the teacher felt the student had attained mastery of the previous one.

Schultz said, "The Western sequence can't be the Eastern sequence. In the West, what we want is abundance of health, abundance of love, abundance of friends. We want abundance of time. In the East, it was a different theory. You were born a Brahmin and that's what you became. 'All is coming' is your evolution, how you want to be, how you want to see eternity, how you want to grow with your community. 'All is coming' is not a black Mercedes. It's not enlightenment. But we do have the power to transform our miserable self into a positive self" (Crooks 2017).

Schultz taught a modified version of classical ashtanga in which he incorporated postures from all of the ashtanga series and allowed students to experiment with the various forms. These classes were some of the first power yoga offerings in the West and the beginnings of the Rocket style of yoga. As a result, Jois called Schultz "the bad man of ashtanga yoga" because of Schultz's interest in teaching second- and third-series poses not yet authorized by Jois (Russel 2018).

In the *Yogi Times* article, Schultz explained his relationship with ashtanga yoga. "I left the ashtanga Mysore system but I still practice ashtanga, I just don't see it like you," he said. "Ashtanga for me is a science of sequencing breath and movement to create an effect. The effect is transformation where you see growth in your life. You see change happening slowly. You see the shell chipping away and a new being emerges. And you learn to take that off the mat" (Crooks 2017).

Schultz was influential in the San Francisco yoga scene of the 1990s and beyond, referring to himself as the Mayor of Folsom Street, the street where his studio, It's Yoga, was located. He was able to bridge the gap between the traditional and the social aspects of yoga, with his studio being a gathering place not just for yoga but also for music, parties, dance, and even social and political movements (Lurrey 2021).

Larry Schultz created three series of postures based on a modification of the classical ashtanga series. For students, these routines renewed energy and vitality in the body by working directly on the joints and stimulating all of the body's systems. For teachers, the routines offered a creative outlet to express themselves honestly in their personal practice, while simultaneously offering an intelligent system of movement based on set sequences that can safely guide all practitioners through the flow of breath and asana.

In the mid-1990s, Schultz was invited to travel on tour with the Grateful Dead as the band's personal yoga teacher, leading the band and their entourage through yoga classes before concerts. While on tour with the Grateful Dead, one of the band members asked Schultz what the name of his yoga was. Schultz replied that it didn't have a name, at which point Bob Weir said, "It should be called Rocket yoga, because it gets you there faster!" And just like that, the name *Rocket* was born.

In an interview in *Deadhead* magazine, Phil Lesh credits Larry Schultz and ashtanga yoga with having a real effect on the music of the tour and giving him personally a new feeling of centeredness (Cushman 1995). Schultz toured with the Grateful Dead, honing and solidifying the Rocket sequences until the death of Jerry Garcia in 1995.

> "The Rocket is designed to wake up the nervous system and feed it the precious prana it craves while promoting a spirit of change and freedom in the practice."
>
> —Larry Schultz

All in all, Schultz created three yoga sequences—referred to as *Rocket I*, *Rocket II*, and *Rocket III*—helping to build the foundation of power yoga. The Rocket routines are a revision of the traditional ashtanga series and destroy the hierarchy of postures and empower practitioners to own their creative process. By following the foundation that the Rocket style provides, they are able to add their own variations while honoring the teachings of traditional ashtanga yoga.

Rocket yoga gets you to a space of happiness and acceptance—a space where your inner voice sings and guides you in the right direction. Schultz designed an asana sequence that invigorates and strengthens students with advanced postures while remaining accessible through modifications and, above all, practicing acceptance of each body's present abilities.

The thread of commitment to sequence that runs through Schultz's personal practice, his trademark Rocket classes, the weekly class schedule, and the widening circle of its yoga studios is clear. "Yoga ultimately is a socialization tool," he said. "First you have to learn it for yourself and love yourself on a day-to-day basis. Then it's about service. The planet wants us to serve each other. We're all miniature versions of Gandhi and Mother Teresa, all those great examples. But most people don't know how to share what they love" (Crooks 2017).

"When yoga came to the West, I had the good fortune to find a great teacher, the best teacher for me, and to grow because of the practice," Schultz said. "A lot of people don't have that. My vision is to have yoga all over the planet and to make it safe and effective" (Crooks 2017).

The Rocket Philosophy

The philosophy of Rocket yoga reveals itself in the practice, reflects back to the old literature such as the *Bhagavad Gita* and the *Yoga Sutras*, and then finds a home in the heart of each student. The way that each student practices, interprets their feelings, and builds their inner home is unique to each individual. Rocket yoga is about your individual journey within. Along with Schultz's philosophy and my personal philosophy, there is room for you to add your own.

"A philosophy gives meaning and purpose to the practice of yoga."

—Larry Schultz

Schultz's Philosophy

The following are tenets that Schultz considered important to his personal yoga philosophy. Your own experiences, the deep questions that you have, and how you interpret the answers will shape your own yoga philosophy over time.

Living in the Question

Questions will arise in your daily practice and through everyday living. It is crucial to learn to listen to that inner voice and to hold on to those questions until answers are revealed.

Practice What You Teach; Teach What You Practice

Pertaining to physical postures in the yoga practice as well as the spiritual aspects of the practice, this can be offering students only yoga poses that teachers have done in their own practice as well as heeding the advice teachers present to students when it comes to tenets for living.

Function Over Form

Bring life into each posture by focusing not on how they look but on how they feel in the body.

Drishti

Most students constantly look outside themselves during practice. Drishti is the practice of a focused gaze during asana practice. By intentionally setting vision to a specific point, one trains the mind to find stillness. When the gaze is turned inward, one's practice, purpose, and creativity unfold.

Control and Surrender

Letting go is how you begin to take control. By acting without attachment to the end results, you are able to live in truth and simplicity.

Nauliland

Ultimately, yoga is about freedom: freeing the mind so that you are able to live in your truth. That freedom is exemplified by *Nauliland*, a term that refers not just to a retreat center in California but also to a state of mind, as explained in the sidebar Understanding Nauliland.

Understanding Nauliland

For Schultz, Nauliland was a pause, a break from modern society's conditioning and standards that allows people to come together and be in the moment: a place to be together, to be on the mat doing the physical yoga practice, and to be in the circle having philosophy talks. It was a place to communicate with each other and create a foundation and a sense of community support that allow people to grab into the real world with a little more stability, direction, drive, and inspiration.

Nauliland is also a physical place that people celebrate as the unification of a community, not unlike a modern-day ashram. From the modern yoga teacher trainings Schultz held in San Francisco to all the yoga studios where people gather now, when people come together and leave behind their social conditioning, their social responsibilities are put on hold momentarily. Placing this retreat in your daily life allows you to honor your path, yourself, your own transformation, and your self-realization. It also allows you to celebrate with those around you. Nauliland is a place you can visit and that you can take with you whenever the community gets together and decides to celebrate together for a certain amount of time.

And when you can't travel to a certain destination, Nauliland is the place inside your heart where yoga resides. For Schultz, it was a place for living life through your heart and through your senses—what you see with your eyes, what you feel with your body, what you hear with your ears—rather than through the mind, which can be clouded and full of judgment and misdirection. Schultz said, "Pay attention to what you see with your eyes open, but know that what you think is make-believe."

What Makes Rocket Yoga Unique?

Although it is rooted in the foundation of ashtanga yoga, three characteristics set the Rocket style apart from other vinyasa flow or power yoga styles.

Versatility

The Rocket sequences are set routines that offer a solid foundation from which creativity can flourish. This creates continuity between Rocket yoga students and teachers worldwide by providing a base sequence that is agreed on. This unique sequencing is a thread that runs through the entire series from standing to seated asanas. From this standardized sequence, optional transitions and additional asanas can be added to offer more detail that is specific to the teacher's chosen physical focus. This makes the Rocket sequences some of the most versatile vinyasa sequences, offering teachers a place to authentically share their strengths and create an experience unique to each student's needs.

Completeness

Considered an all-inclusive practice, Rocket yoga breaks through common areas of tension, habitual patterns, and energy blockages to combat one's tendencies toward stagnancy and resistance in the body. Grounding forward folds are balanced by expansive backbends. Handstands and arm balance variations keep the energy levels high and encourage students to connect to their inner power and shift their perspective. Spinal twisting, hip openers, and core-strengthening exercises create a well-balanced and uplifting sequence of postures. Rocket yoga has gained global recognition as a complete, feel-good practice that challenges the student, opens the body, and clears the mind.

Accessibility

Rocket yoga introduces the vigorous practice of ashtanga yoga to the masses by providing a standard class format and allowing access to the benefits of the ashtanga postures without requiring feats of flexibility or strength. Poses are offered by the teacher according to each student's abilities, not the rigid hierarchy of poses in classical ashtanga. Accessible to all levels, the Rocket style provides modifications to beginners and variations that challenge even the most advanced students, allowing the benefits to be felt by all.

My Personal Yoga Philosophy

Many of Schultz's personal philosophies resonate with me. However, years of personal practice have brought to light the following personal truths that guide my own practice as a teacher and as a student in this lineage.

Yoga Practice Is Designed to Teach You About Yourself

I strive to create and provide a space for each practitioner to express and grow in their personal practice in order to achieve this goal of self-discovery. I offer freedom inside their practice and focus my attention on aiding them in developing discipline and strength for their mind and body.

From here, I believe that each practitioner will develop at their individual pace in a safe and effective manner. I teach what I practice and say what I feel: grace, comfort, acceptance, and love.

> "We do the practice to love ourselves so we can learn to love others more."
>
> —Larry Schultz

Health Is Freedom

By allowing ourselves to connect with how we feel, we learn how to control and how to create from a space that is calm, clear, and focused. Through yoga asana, we create and control the level of health inside our body, mind, and soul through the feelings that arise while we practice. Once our mind is at ease and our attention is focused, we are able to cleanse and purify all blocks and create a blank slate from which we begin to manifest our deepest desires and then learn to let them go. This practice brings health, which is happiness, and happiness is one of our most important goals.

Free Agency Is a Gift

For every type of person, there is a different kind of yoga, and for every desired effect, there is a sequence of actions to create it. We are all given the gift to choose what resonates with us best. Choice is a powerful tool—so we must use it wisely. The best students question their teachers and require proof through personal experience before they give their trust to a philosophy. We must all become scientists of our own reality, and by recognizing this power of choice, we are left with only a smile knowing that wherever we are, it's because we chose to be there.

Developing Your Own Yoga Philosophy

A yoga philosophy is a framework that supports your intentions and goals as a student and a teacher. This philosophy will be strengthened over time through personal experience and by seeking truths that resonate with you. Establishing a personal philosophy that inspires and influences your lifestyle is a practice within itself that will keep your values and intentions clear.

Developing your philosophy may take time. Allow your ideas to percolate over time and be open to changing your philosophy as you learn new things about yourself. Actively seek new experiences to help you see things from different perspectives. Listen to your own inner teacher, and commit to nurturing your philosophy daily.

Ask yourself the following questions to guide you, and then write your own yoga philosophy in the space provided.

What do you do to practice yoga each day?

On the best of days, what does practicing yoga give you?

On the worst of days, what does practicing yoga give you?

How can you share your personal yoga practice with others?

If you are training as a teacher, ask yourself the following questions to guide your teaching philosophy, and then write your answers about your philosophy in the space provided.

Who do you want to teach?

How do you want to teach?

Where do you want to teach?

When do you want to teach?

Why do you want to teach?

_____

_____

_____

_____

_____

_____

_____

_____

_____

The Fundamentals

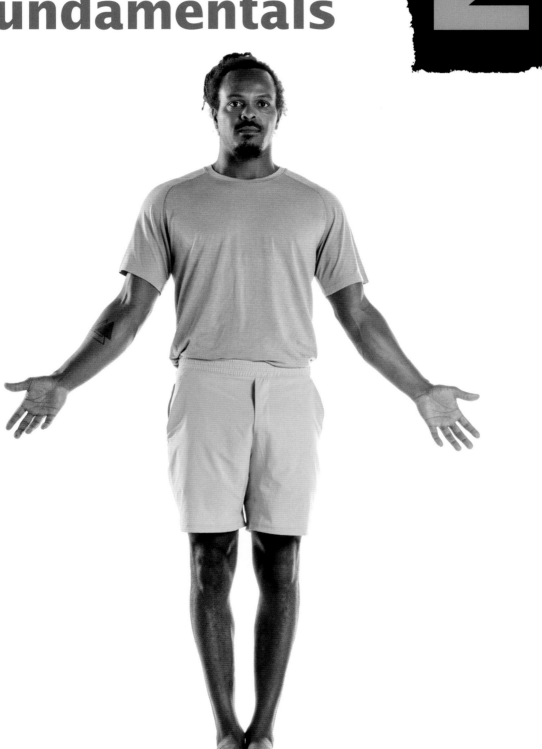

2

Before you dive into a full practice, it is helpful to know the foundational elements—that is, what the practice is built on. When everything else is stripped away, what are the essential parts we are left with? These fundamentals form the backbone of your practice. Together with your own diligence and commitment to your craft, they unlock the full benefits of this yoga practice.

Introduction to the Tristhana Method

Classical ashtanga yoga and Rocket yoga are both built on the tristhana, meaning three folds or three parts. Tristhana comprises the three foundational attributes that distinguish classical ashtanga yoga from other types of hatha yoga and provide a road map for safely practicing asanas, or placing one's body into a certain shape. The three attributes of tristhana are breath, focused gaze, and accessing an energetic lock in a specific posture. In Sanskrit, these are known as pranayama, drishti, and bandha.

Asanas alone are not yoga and will not deliver the full transformative power of a yoga practice. Without all three attributes working in unison, there would be no vinyasa involved with the yoga. Vinyasa is the intentional linking of breath and movement, a concept we will dive deeper into in chapter 3. However, when a pose is combined with a specific gazing point and a particular quality of breath, the full benefits of yoga can be felt. The tristhana method offers safety within the physical practice and direct progression on the path of self-realization through the purification of the three bodies: physical, mental, and spiritual. Here, we take a closer look at each of these qualities.

Pranayama, or Breath

Pranayama is the idea of expanding, controlling, and directing one's prana, which is life force or vitality. The beginner's point of introduction to pranayama, the concept of expanding and controlling one's life force energy, is best done with breath control and retention. However, it is not only these breathing techniques that create the expansion and control of prana. The practices of posture, a focused gaze, and breath control together provide the expansion of prana.

It is the movement of breathing that easily connects us to the idea of movement creating life. Without breath, we would surely die. So the movement of the breath is essential to life like the beating of the heart is. Our bodies and minds are external parts of this existence, just like our

> "When the Breath wanders, the mind is unsteady, but when the Breath is still, so is the mind still."
>
> —*Hatha Yoga Pradipika*

cars, televisions, and radios. Our cars and TVs need fuel or electricity to function. Prana is the fuel or wave that carries the signal of life through the body and mind. This signal moves us and manifests itself in many forms from physical movements to thought waves. Where there is movement, there is this life force. Prana is the catalyst for life when it infuses movement into the body and even the subtlest movements in the thoughts of the mind. Pranayama is not just moving the breath but also controlling the movements in the body that produce the breath and controlling the subtleties of the thought that is behind the breath.

In your practice it is important to work with your respiratory system to its fullest capacity and function. Learning how to control your breath requires an intimate connection to all the stages of the breath and how they affect the body and mind. There are many breathing exercises that yoga practitioners use for many different effects. However, only one breathing technique specifically aids your practice of ashtanga yoga and Rocket vinyasa. This is the ujjayi breath. This technique is also useful for other vinyasa-type practices, so it can be seen as a universal breathing principle for vinyasa practice.

Ujjayi is translated as "victorious." This particular breathing technique can be done on its own in a comfortable seated position, or it can be applied consciously and with great intention during the practice of your vinyasa. Ujjayi breathing is a beginner technique. Even so, it can have a powerful and profound effect on your body. The qualities that define the ujjayi make observing the breath easier for both the student and the teacher. More awareness of the breath will lead to a fuller experience in the yoga practice. Ujjayi breathing also creates a safer experience because the breath will inform you of whether you are overexerting yourself physically or whether there is still room to push your edge. The three main qualities of the ujjayi breath are rhythm, sound, and movement.

Rhythm

Breathing is rhythmic. Inhalations and exhalations should be done with the same timing. A five-second inhalation requires a five-second exhalation. If a yoga pose is difficult and causes the breath to lose its rhythm, then the breath control is lost. If the breath is without control, then there is no yoga. Postures should be modified as needed to maintain the desired rhythm of the breath.

Sound

The sound of the breath is smooth. All sound comes from the constriction of the throat. A smooth hissing sound like the wind or waves of the ocean is the intention. This sound brings a meditative and calming quality to the breath. Similar to rhythm, sound enables you to quickly discern whether you are physically overexerting yourself. Difficulty maintaining the sound of the ujjayi breath is your signal to find more ease in the posture.

Movement

The breath's movement during an inhalation is an expansion as well as a lifting of the chest and rib cage. On the exhalation, the core contracts and squeezes into the spine. Each breath should create an obvious shift and change in the body's posture. This is not a normal breath. It is an excited or active breath that provides a deep, continuous feed of oxygen, or prana, and movement to the body.

Drishti, or Focused Gaze

A steady gaze leads to a steady mind. Drishti is seen both in a physical and a metaphysical way. It is not only literally what you see but also an intentional observation of the inner workings of nature. It is where you are physically gazing at the moment as well as your intention for your practice. Nine physical drishti points are traditionally used in the asana practice. Rocket yoga offers other options beyond these nine points when creating variations, but these will serve as your basic alignments during your practice. These are the nine drishti points:

1. *Nasikagra*—tip of the nose
2. *Bhrumadhya*—between the eyebrows (third eye)
3. *Nabhi chakra*—navel
4. *Hastagrai*—hand or fingertips
5. *Padhayoragrai*—toes
6. *Parshva*—to the right
7. *Parshva*—to the left
8. *Angustha ma dyai*—thumb
9. *Urdhva or antara*—up to the sky

The drishti establishes a sense of balance in the spine. The direction of your gaze affects the position of the head and neck, which will determine the alignment of your yoga asana. Pay attention to the specific drishti point for each asana in chapters 4 to 7. Where the eyes go, energy flows.

The direction and fixed gaze of your eyes also brings an intense concentration over your practice. The eyes provide the sense of sight, which can be a distraction when they are focused on external processes. Your gaze must turn inward for introspection to take place. By holding the gaze on a specific place, you start to turn the senses inward and increase the sensitivity and skill of the action at hand. The same works with focusing the mind to think only of the duty or action that is taking place and keeping it from wandering to other thoughts, places, or dreams. Through proper intention, you see beyond the physical realm and into a deep image of the self.

Your gaze also relates to your memory and your dreams—the vision you have of the past and for the future. As a yoga practitioner, you understand that truth lies in the present moment, the eternal now. It is not found in the past, in memories of things that are no more. And it is not found in your dreams of realizing what you imagine you will desire in the future. Reality is only in the present. Through focused drishti, you keep yourself involved with the present moment. You commit to being here now. Once you are firmly grounded in the present moment, you will have a point from which to move forward. You will be able to manifest your dreams through focused intention—through your drishti. This is the secret. Your mind will attract what it is focused on. Even without physically moving the body through different yoga postures, you can cultivate focus and learn to use your drishti in meditation.

One way to improve vision, memory, and focus is to practice trataka, which is a meditation technique that involves gazing at the flame of a candle. If you don't have a candle, you can also gaze at any object, such as a flower. For these instructions, we will use a candle.

Prepare and Practice

Preparation

Set up a candle in a dark or dimly lit room. The candle should be about two feet (61 cm) away from you and about chest high. Find a comfortable place to sit. The room should have no draft or wind that would cause the candle to flicker. A still flame is best.

Practice

Gaze at the tip of the candle intently for 10 to 15 seconds or until you feel you can no longer hold your gaze (see figure), then close your eyes. With your eyes closed, you will see the afterimage of the flame in your mind's eye. Concentrate on this image. Begin to envision the qualities of the object—color, smell, touch, and its entire essence. As the image fades, allow it to slowly disappear and then slowly open your eyes. Repeat the exercise.

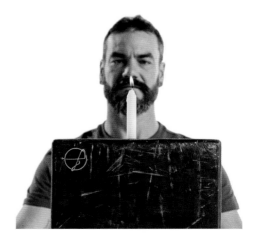

Try not to look elsewhere in the room as you do this. Do your best to focus your drishti completely on the object. At the end of the meditation, make a note of how you feel. This practice helps develop concentration and understanding of the object being meditated on.

Trataka is not dangerous, but it should be done with caution if you have glaucoma, epilepsy, schizophrenia, or migraines. It should not be performed if you are feeling angry, anxious, or agitated or have a headache because it can worsen these experiences.

Bandhas, or Energetic Locks

Bandhas are energy locks, or valves, that help control the flow of prana in our nadis. Nadis are energetic lines, or passages, that run through the body in a pattern similar to our nervous system; more will be explained about the relationship between the bandhas and nadis later in this section. The three main bandhas applied in classical ashtanga as well as in Rocket yoga are all located along the centerline of the body (see figure 2.1). They correspond to the three diaphragms within the body:

1. *Mula bandha (root lock)*—pelvic girdle
2. *Uddiyana bandha (abdominal lock)*—diaphragm
3. *Jalandhara bandha (throat lock)*—voice box

More than these three main bandhas can be used to understand the function of bandha both for internal and external control. For example, the hasta bandha is a great visual example as the open hand closes into a fist. This shows an area closing in on itself to centralize all the power into one place. The feet and most joints, like shoulders and knees, can also use bandhas for protection and stabilization. However, we will focus here on the three main bandhas.

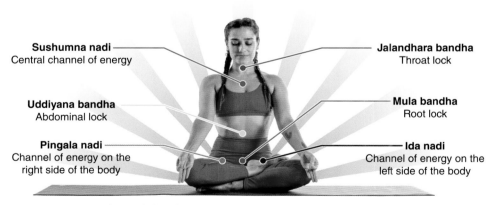

Sushumna nadi — Central channel of energy

Jalandhara bandha — Throat lock

Uddiyana bandha — Abdominal lock

Mula bandha — Root lock

Pingala nadi — Channel of energy on the right side of the body

Ida nadi — Channel of energy on the left side of the body

Figure 2.1   Nadis and the three bandhas.

To understand how bandhas work, think of a river with dams. When the dams are open, water rushes freely down the river. When a dam is closed, the energy of the river can be transformed into electrical energy. Ideally, the river should be full and freely flowing, and the dams should be able to lock or unlock without trouble, harnessing energy when it's needed.

Similarly, prana is the flow of energy inside the body. When the prana is flowing freely through the nadis, the body is at its optimal state of health. In yoga, it is believed that prana is in a constant state of flowing in and out of the body. Controlling the bandhas allows you to capture the prana inside to increase your prana and flush it through all of the nadis to awaken the spiritual body. Practice allows for the use of the bandhas to push the prana up the sushumna to the next highest chakra, purifying and curing ailments and imbalances that lie along the way.

Bandhas have a direct connection with the energetic body within, but it is easier to describe bandhas in physical terms through the muscles and organs that correspond with them. Some systems of yoga only see bandhas as a subtle energetic process. We will move from the gross to the subtle by allowing the bandha to reflect a physical muscle contraction or group of muscle contractions that cause the simultaneous internal relaxation to open particular energetic areas of the body.

Through practice and increased sensitivity, which result from the purification of the energetic body, this action of bandhas becomes more and more subtle and constant without much effort at all. The idea of contracting a bandha causes an internal opening of that area like a lotus flower bud being squeezed from the bottom and opening its petals.

The bandhas can be practiced together or individually at specific times during asana, pranayama, mudra, visualization, meditation practice, and cleansing kriyas, which are discussed at the end of this chapter. They also occur spontaneously, especially in children, but also in yogis who can allow themselves to be moved by the evolutionary transformational force—the kundalini. There are many more bandhas than the classic three acknowledged in ashtanga vinyasa, but some do not have outward flows and, therefore, we do not need to practice those bandhas, or if we did, there would be little effect. Our goal is to focus on the three bandhas that help to untie the knots that restrict our natural flow of energy up the sushumna.

When starting a yoga practice, there is no need to focus on the bandhas. Start with learning the gross movements and placements for each pose, and add in a calm and steady breath while holding the pose. Only after you are able to perform each pose with a stable breath should you focus on the subtle energetics of the bandhas.

The Chakras

In the ashtanga system we acknowledge the subtle body, the energetic centers and channels within the physical body. The seven chakras are located along the spine from the crown of the head to the base of the sacrum (see figure 2.2). *Chakra* is a Sanskrit word meaning "wheel" or "cycle." Each chakra has its own characteristics, vibrational frequency, color, and associated element.

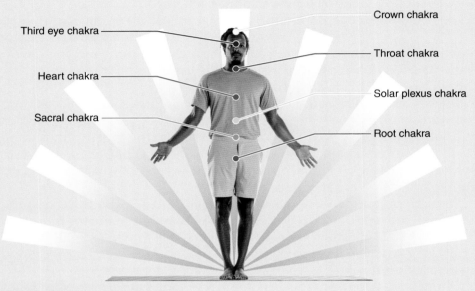

Figure 2.2 The seven chakras.

Although the chakras cannot be seen or touched, their impact can be felt both physically and emotionally when they are open or blocked. The most common and basic description of the chakra system is outlined below.

Name	Location	Color	Element	Associated ashtanga limb	Governs
Crown chakra, or sahasrara (thousand petal white lotus)	Crown of the head	White	Cosmos	Dyana and samadhi	Connection to the cosmos, individual dissolves into universal consciousness, enlightenment
Third eye chakra, or ajna (unlimited authority)	Third eye or forehead	Violet or indigo	Light	Dharana	Illusion of separateness and duality ceases, intuition and creativity, right hemisphere receptive mode of consciousness

Name	Location	Color	Element	Associated ashtanga limb	Governs
Throat chakra, or vishuddha (pure)	Throat	Blue	Sound	Pratyahara	Verbal communication, logical, linear thought, left hemisphere active mode of consciousness
Heart chakra, or anahata (unstricken or liberated)	Heart, center of the chest	Green	Air	Pranayama	Agape (unconditional love), compassion, healing, breathing
Solar plexus chakra, or manipura (city of gems)	Navel to solar plexus	Yellow	Fire	Asana	Power, physical strength, belongingness
Sacral chakra, or svadhisthana (dwelling place of the self)	Uddiyana bandha	Orange	Water	Niyamas	Generative, procreation, emotions
Root chakra, or muladhara (foundation or root)	Mula bandha or perineum (for men)	Red	Earth	Yamas	Grounding and personal security, connection to the earth

Mula Bandha

Associated Chakra: Muladhara chakra

Benefits

Strengthens the pelvic floor muscles

Relieves menstrual pain

Lowers blood pressure

Stabilizes the pelvis to allow for more mobility in the spine

Provides a feeling of lightness and integration

Calms the nervous system

Cleanses the muladhara chakra

Contraindications

Pregnancy

Hypertension

Anxiety

Cardiovascular issues

Hernia

Peptic ulcers

The root (mula) lock moves the earth energy up through the muladhara chakra (root chakra) system, connecting above it to the water chakra (swadhisthana), while also serving as the valve connecting sky energy, or spirit, below it to the center of the earth. Mula bandha keeps the energy flowing between the body and the earth.

The muladhara chakra is the most important chakra in hatha, kundalini, and tantric yoga as well as the most mysterious. It is where our dormant potential and animal power reside, and it is from here the kundalini is activated and enters into the central channel (sushumna), activating the superconscious network. This is not an archaic myth or fantasy and should not be ignored nor demeaned, but rather it is knowledge essential to success in hatha yoga. Mula bandha is designed to keep this energy flowing in this region. In yogic literature, the goddess Kundalini is pictured as lying dormant in the muladhara chakra in the form of a serpent coiled three and a half times around a lingam (a sacred Hindu object representing the god Shiva). The symbol for this chakra is a downward-facing triangle normally, but when the chakra is activated (by an activated kundalini) the triangle points upward.

Prepare and Practice

Preparation

The best preparation for mula bandha is ashwini mudra in order to tone the nerves, glands, and muscles of the area. Ashwini mudra, horse gesture, is the rhythmic contracting and relaxing of the anal sphincter. It can be done lying supine with the legs at 90 degrees or in a simple and comfortable seat.

Practice

Contract the anal sphincter muscle and hold for as long as you can before releasing. For men it is the upward turning (like a triangle) of the space about one inch (2.5 cm) above the perineum. The perineal space becomes indented, domed, or sucked in and up, creating empty space for the front of the pubic bone and sacrum to move toward each other. It is sometimes described as the sensation of cutting off the flow of urine. It is similar for women, except that the center of the action occurs at the cervix being drawn up and in. This is not a pelvic tilt (anterior or posterior, which occurs between the humerus and pelvis or between the trunk and pelvis), but rather mula bandha occurs deep within the moveable elements and energetic dynamics of the pelvic girdle itself. It is an energy dynamic more than a muscle movement. The sensation here is similar to performing a Kegel. Perform this 8 to 10 times.

Uddiyana Bandha

Associated Chakra: Manipura chakra (solar plexus chakra)

Benefits

Relieves constipation and indigestion

Strengthens the abdominal muscles and diaphragm

Increases blood flow in the abdomen and blood flow to the brain

Stimulates gastric fire

Connects the upper and lower body to work as a whole

Opens blockages in the manipura chakra, connecting the water center (swadhisthana chakra) with the air center (anahata chakra)

Helps untie vishnu granthi

Contraindications

Stomach or intestinal distress or ulcers

Hernia

High blood pressure

Heart disease

Glaucoma

Pregnancy

Uddiyana means "flying upward." It is the bandha that moves the energy upward from the earth, water, and fire centers into the heart (air) chakra, strongly influencing the efficacy of the lower bandhas by "making room" on top. Some practitioners say that it helps suck the energy into the central column. It prevents tension and stagnation to develop or accumulate in the navel region. Uddiyana bandha not only cleanses the region around the navel and the front of the lower spine, but it also purifies and energizes the entire body.

Prepare and Practice

Preparation

Tadagi mudra (tank seal) is a simple pose that offers an approximation of the engagement of uddiyana bandha. By lying down, you can use the force of gravity to assist in finding the right engagement. To assume this pose, lie flat on your back and extend the arms overhead until the backs of the hands touch the ground. Reach the arms away from your center as much as possible. At the same time, reach the heels away from the body. You are stretching in opposite directions. As you are stretching, allow the belly to contract into the torso. Breathe normally in this position, allowing the lower belly to remain hollow throughout the breath.

(continued)

(continued)

Practice

Although *uddiyana* means "flying upward," this term refers to the energy, not the navel point, which remains downward and back toward the spine. For best results and especially to first learn the effects, start by standing with the feet approximately shoulder-width apart and facing forward. Take one hand to the back to feel the part of the spine that lines up opposite the navel, which will be near the top of the lumbar curve approximately at T12 (this spot on the spine will vary according to individuals, seasons, and conditions). Loosen the area in the back and visualize the navel moving inward toward it, without the spine moving away from the navel. Do not hunch the shoulders or collapse the chest by concentrating the movement at the solar plexus and below.

Next, bend the knees slightly, and place the hands on the inside of the lower thighs with the meat of the palms resting on the top of the lower thighs and fingers pointing slightly in toward the knees. Avoid placing undue weight on the hands, arms, or shoulders. Avoid torquing the knees or legs, rounding the shoulders, and collapsing the upper torso or upper back. Let the top of the scapula sink away from the ears as the heart remains lifted. The tailbone moves toward the pubic bone, allowing the tailbone and sacrum to sink down and find the mula bandha. Resist the tendency of the pelvis to round in retroversion or tuck in anteversion; keep it long and stable in mula bandha.

Here, take a deep breath in through your nose, then exhale quickly and forcibly also through your nose (or pursed lips) as you contract your abdominals to push as much air as possible out of your lungs. Then relax your abdominal muscles completely. Perform a mock inhalation by expanding your rib cage (thorax) as if you were going to inhale, but don't actually take any air in. You only want to physically expand the rib cage. The expansion of the rib cage without air creates a vacuum effect that pulls the abdominal muscles and viscera up into the thorax and hollows the belly. Hold for 5 to 10 seconds, then slowly release and take a full breath. Repeat for 3 to 10 rounds.

Jalandhara Bandha

Associated Chakra: Vishuddhi chakra (throat chakra)

Benefits

Improves breath retention capacity

Develops the ability to concentrate

Improves thyroid function

Stabilizes metabolism

Contraindications

Hypertension

Neck pain

Upper-back pain

Cardiovascular problems

Vertigo

Cervical spondylitis

Untreated thyroid problems

The throat lock's purpose is to compress the neck or, more specifically, the upper-esophageal sphincter. This compression increases the flow of prana in the upper chest and to the brain. This bandha is not usually fully engaged while doing asanas but instead is a soft constriction. It is only fully engaged when in meditation or during the finishing poses of a full practice.

Prepare and Practice

Preparation

Jalandhara bandha is the easiest of the bandhas to access. Simply find a comfortable seat with no distractions.

Practice

From a comfortable seat, lightly place the hands on top of your lap or knees. Take a full breath in, then draw the center of the sternum forward to meet your chin. Allow the chin to drop inward and downward just enough to touch the chest. This movement should elongate the back of the neck and soften the throat. Keep the shoulders down and the remainder of the body relaxed. Hunching the shoulders forward to get the chin to rest on the sternum will not create the benefits of jalandhara bandha. Hold your breath for as long as you can. Release the bandha by lifting the chin. It is important to release the bandha before exhaling. Repeat for 3 to 10 cycles.

Rather than conceptualizing the bandha as bringing the chin in toward the sternal arch, it might be easier to visualize it as bringing the sternal arch up to meet the chin. Visualize making a double chin by moving the heart forward, sinking the scapula, and moving the chin down and slightly back.

Maha Bandha

The three classic bandhas, mula bandha, uddiyana bandha, and jalandhara bandha, when practiced together are called maha bandha, or tribandha. Only a few poses require all three to be applied simultaneously. During your asana practice, maha bandha promotes constant awareness of the internal support and processes at a cellular and energetic level. This allows the energy to build all the way to the end of the practice where it is released at the moment of meditation and rest. Maha bandha is powerful when done correctly. The precautions for each individual bandha also apply when practicing maha bandha.

Prepare and Practice

Preparation

Setu bandhasana (bridge pose) is a good pose for starting to feel the engagement of maha bandha without excessive effort. Lie flat on your back and bend your knees, placing your feet flat on the ground, hip-width apart. Arms are long by your side.

Practice

In this position, inhale deeply, then on an exhale, press the arms and feet down into the ground and lift the hips as high as possible (see figure). Bring the hands to the lower back to support the hips, if needed. You can also place a block under the sacrum for a more restorative effect. Feel the abdominals gravitate toward the thoracic cavity, opening the base of the rib cage. Allow them to move with gravity. Stay here for 5 to10 breaths. Notice how all three bandhas are engaged: mula bandha through the lower abdominal tone, uddiyana bandha through the opening of the lower ribs and the gravitational force on the inner abdomen, and jalandhara bandha associated with the cervical flexion of the neck.

To feel the engagement of maha bandha even more strongly, from setu bandhasana, fully exhale all the breath. During the pause after the exhalation, slowly begin to lower the spine toward the ground. You will feel a natural lift in the pelvic floor as the contents of the abdominal cavity move toward the vacuum of the thoracic space. This is the sensation of maha bandha.

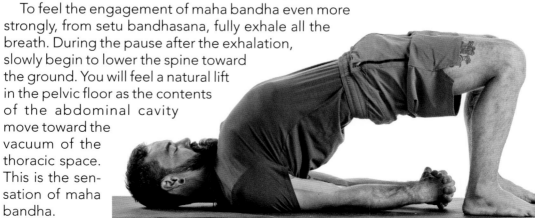

Finding the Bandhas

The practices of certain kriyas (yogic cleansing techniques) are a great exercise for bandha awareness. Nauli kriya is the most important kriya for the beginner yogi to learn and perform and can help to access the uddiyana bandha. This exercise is said to cure diseases in the abdominal region and encourages a healthy digestive system. It should be done on an empty stomach and preferably in the morning before eating. It can be incorporated into your daily cleansing activities like brushing your teeth, taking a shower, and yoga asana. To perform this exercise, follow these steps:

1. Stand with the feet slightly wider than the hips, then bend the knees.
2. Place the hands on top of the knees with the fingers turned inward to spread the scapula apart and broaden the upper back. Round the spine by tucking the tailbone slightly and encouraging the abdominal region to relax and soften.
3. Look toward your belly to observe the movements. Exhale all the air from the body, leaving the lungs completely empty.
4. Draw the diaphragm and organs up into the rib cage area as you expand and stretch the rib cage (see figure a). This is called bahya kumbhaka. By taking advantage of the atmospheric pressure that surrounds us and the void that is left in the body from the kumbhaka, an internal vacuum is created that aids in the manipulation of the internal body. This vacuum creates a deep internal massage and energetic stimulations when the lower abdominal region lifts.
5. Maintaining the vacuum and lift in the abdomen, try to move the abdominal muscles in and out or from one side to the other (see figures b and c). If you have difficulty creating the vacuum in the thoracic cavity, try to strongly push the palms of the hands down into the upper thighs. Pushing the femur bones down will naturally create a slight hollowing of the lower abdomen.

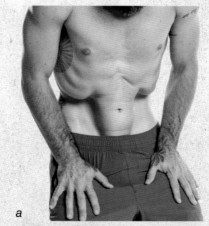

a

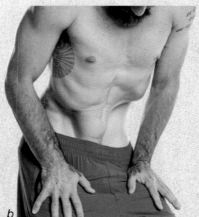

b

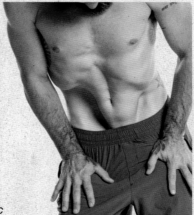

c

Daily Cleansing Rituals

Cleansing rituals are not specific to yoga. Many cleansing rituals are already part of our daily activities in society. Taking baths and showers to clean the skin and brushing our teeth make us feel clean and fresh. This affects our well-being and prepares us for our day. Yogic cleansing techniques were specifically designed for the hatha yogi. They were originally suggested for all who practice asana and pranayama to prepare the physical and subtle bodies with the shatkarma, the six cleansing techniques.

1. *Jala neti*—cleansing of the nasal passages by pouring filtered water through the nose
2. *Agnisara dhauti*—cleansing of the digestive tract
3. *Vasti*—cleansing of the colon through the use of an enema
4. *Trataka*—purifying through gazing at a fixed point or the flame of a candle
5. *Nauli*—cleansing of the abdominal organs through specific muscular engagement
6. *Kapalabhati*—removing toxins from the body through a breathing technique

When practiced in full, the shatkarma can be intense and require training because some of the methods can be dangerous if done without proper guidance. Some kriyas require a particular apparatus, such as a neti pot—a small container with a spout used for rinsing the nasal passages with saline solution. These practices are usually done within the privacy of the home, the same as regular bathing and cleaning practices. Vasti, or enemas, are not part of Rocket yoga; although under the guidance of a professional, they can be good for alleviating many common ailments in the digestion and elimination processes.

Only the purification techniques that are accessible as a daily ritual done by oneself are focused on here. In Rocket yoga, these daily cleansing techniques are a preparatory series called the four purifications. Each purification technique can be done alone to great benefit. It is necessary to establish a repetitive practice over 40 days to see the full effects of each pranayama. The four purifications are nadi shodhana pranayama, kapalabhati pranayama, agnisara dhauti, and ashwini mudra.

Nadi Shodhana Pranayama

Nadi shodhana pranayama is a nerve-cleansing technique consisting of simple alternating nostril breathing. This practice evens the breath that enters each nostril, alleviating congestion. It also balances the sympathetic and parasympathetic nervous systems by alternately engaging each one in rhythm until they are used equally.

Prepare and Practice

Preparation

Find a comfortable seated position so all of your attention is on the experience of the breath.

Practice

Start with a pinch-type grip, and use the thumb of your right hand for the right nostril and the ring finger of the same hand for the left nostril. Keep your pointing and middle fingers softly closed into the palm (see figure a). Exhale all the air out through both nostrils. Close the right nostril with the thumb, and inhale through the left side (see figure b). Close the left side with the ring finger (see figure c), then release the thumb from the right nostril and exhale through the right side (see figure d). Then inhale back through the right side. Close the right side with the thumb, then release the ring finger from the left nostril and exhale through the left side. This can initially be performed for about 10 rounds. Build up to 27 rounds (108 breaths). Eventually with focus you can perform 40 rounds or more.

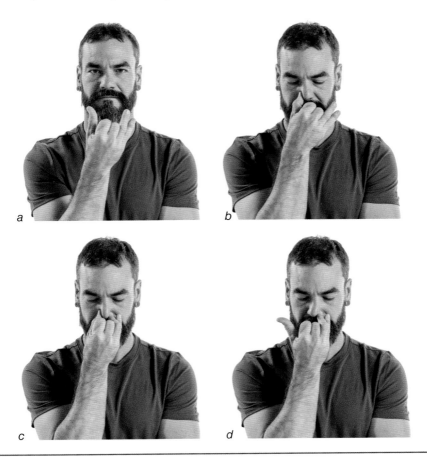

a

b

c

d

Kapalabhati Pranayama

Kapalabhati pranayama is known as the *skull shining breath*. It brings a glow to the forehead of the practitioner as it builds a rising energy and sense of heat that makes the forehead sweat. This is also considered one of the shatkarma techniques. This technique focuses on the action of exhalation only. Rhythmic exhalations are short and sharp, and the inhalation is a natural, effortless refilling of the lungs. People with high blood pressure or lung disease should not practice this pranayama because breathing in this way slightly increases the blood pressure during the exercise.

Prepare and Practice

Preparation

Sit comfortably with the spine erect.

Practice

Take one full breath cycle, exhaling completely. On the next inhale, breathe in only about 60 percent. Use the abdominals and diaphragm to push the air out on the exhalation. After the squeeze of the diaphragm and push of the abdominals into the spine that are associated with the exhalation, relax. This will cause a small amount of air to enter the lungs. Take 30 forced, rhythmic exhalations, and then rest. These can be done rapidly or as slowly as one exhalation per second. Three rounds are efficient to feel the effects. Over time you can build up to 60 breaths and 10 rounds.

Agnisara Dhauti

Agnisara dhauti is translated as "fire wash." This is a technique that requires you to hold your breath as you exercise the function of the diaphragm. This exercise can build an intense heat inside that purifies and cleanses like a low fever. Knowledge and practice of uddiyana bandha will make this exercise most effective.

Prepare and Practice

Preparation

Find a comfortable seated position and look toward the belly.

Practice

Exhale all your breath and hold for the duration of the round. Use the action of your diaphragm to pull the belly up and under the rib cage. The rib cage should expand in all directions. This is often described as a fake inhalation, where you perform the action of inhalation without letting the air come in. The result is a vacuum effect on the torso. Repeat this rhythmically as long as you can with the breath held. Start with 50 pumps over three to five rounds. Eventually you can build up to 100 or even 500 pumps of the belly to stoke the inner fire!

Ashwini Mudra

Ashwini mudra is called the horse mudra. This is an excellent preparatory practice for creating more awareness of the pelvic floor. This exercise is great for beginning the process of mula bandha practice.

Prepare and Practice

Preparation

Sit comfortably with your spine erect.

Practice

Take a deep inhalation and hold the breath for as long as you feel comfortable. Repeatedly with steady rhythm, contract and release the sphincter muscle. During the contraction, feel a pull up and into the base of the spine. Relax, and do not push out. Do this 20 to 60 times per round and build up to 10 rounds.

Advanced Application of the Purifications

An advanced technique is to perform the four purifications together in one routine. The purifications are done in order with no resting breaths between. This brings efficiency to the purification routine because it can be done in a shorter amount of time with the same benefits. Perform this before you begin your asana practice in order to clear your body and mind.

Perform five rounds of nadi shodhana followed by kapalabhati for one round, finishing off with an exhalation retention for agnisara dhauti. Pump as long as you can comfortably hold the breath. Immediately take an inhalation retention and practice ashwini mudra for as long as comfortable. After completing, you can repeat and build up to five rounds. Over time, increase the number of rounds in each purification.

The Progressive Ashtanga Vinyasa Method

3

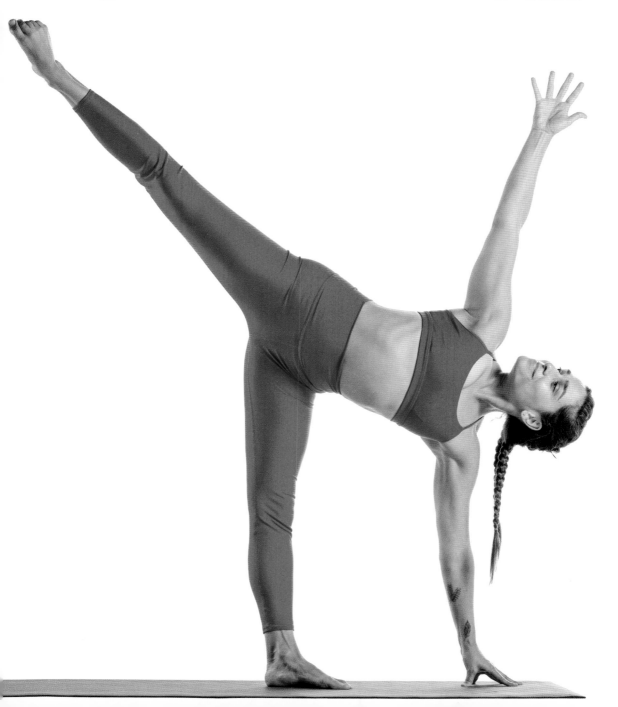

Classical ashtanga is a beautiful but physically demanding practice that can be seen as overly rigid and monotonous. Rocket yoga is a dynamic sequence based on ashtanga yoga that creates more space for exploration and provides more modifications for those who need them. When practiced together, they deliver the benefits of both. On one hand, you are able to see the progression of a pose because you consistently practice in the same way. On the other hand, you have a structure that allows for more playfulness and curiosity. Together, they form the progressive ashtanga vinyasa method—a yoga practice that combines series from both classical ashtanga and Rocket to offer a weekly schedule proven to accelerate your yoga practice.

Introducing the Vinyasa

The Sanskrit word *vinyasa* is translated as "to place in a special way." This implies the need for concentration and awareness of the action within the present moment. In the yoga practice, vinyasa refers to the union of breath and body, moving together with intention. It is this union that forms the foundation of classical ashtanga as well as Rocket yoga. The following are the defining characteristics of the vinyasa technique that will be the basis of your yoga practice.

Presence

The vinyasa technique keeps you in the present. Ideally, this works by keeping your attention on each movement and breath at that very moment—perfecting each movement along the way so the mind is not distracted by what has passed or what will come. By connecting each movement to a specific breath, it becomes possible to stay in the present moment even through challenging physical movements. Instead of focusing on the tension in the body, bringing the mind to concentrate on the expansiveness of the breath at each moment holds the mind in a state of presence.

Counting

Simple rules can be observed when following a vinyasa practice. A vinyasa system is also a counting system, so it can be viewed with the precision of a mathematical system. Inhalations are always odd numbers and exhalations are always even numbers (for example: movement one—inhale; movement two—exhale; movement three—inhale; movement four—exhale). Sun salutations always begin with an inhalation, extending the arms upward on the first count. Subsequent sun salutations also start on the count of one.

Although classical ashtanga counts each movement and breath aloud, it is not necessary to do so in Rocket yoga. Focus instead on the gross physical movements, the small details of alignment, and the energetic qualities of each posture. For example, inhalations are expansive movements that extend upward, lengthen the body, and untwist. Exhalations are contracting movements that move downward and inward and twist. By following these simple rules, you can create simple and effective vinyasa sequences that follow a breath and energy consciousness.

Transitions

Transitions refer to how you move from one pose to the next. Some transitions need only one breath, and others require more. Classical ashtanga uses the transition that offers the most efficient movement from one pose to the next, linking each movement to a precise breath. Rocket yoga invites you to add difficulty to the transition when possible, releasing the rigidity of a precise breath and allowing for more playfulness in these spaces of movement.

Meditative Movement

The vinyasa absorbs you into a trancelike state. Vinyasa can also be described as the process of transcending from one point of existence to another. The vinyasa is whatever helps you accomplish this process.

Many qualities are carried through this amazing and organic way to create a connection between your physical, mental, and energetic selves. You can begin to understand the science of the breath behind the traditional systems. This gives vinyasa a more specific definition and allows you, no matter the yoga style, to observe the same simple rules of practice.

Precise Placement

A stable foundation is the key to building a stable structure. When force is properly balanced and evenly distributed, the foundation easily provides support for long periods of time. However, if the foundation is damaged or force is unevenly distributed, the structure is exposed to extra strain, which compromises stability and leaves the structure vulnerable. Either slowly or quickly, the structure gives in to gravity and collapses. These principles of architecture can also be applied to the practice of yoga asana. The following exercise provides insight into the structure and alignment needed to properly perform specific yoga asanas.

The body is split into three planes of movement: sagittal, transverse, and coronal. The sagittal plane splits the body into two sides—right and left; the transverse plane splits the body into upper and lower; and the coronal plane splits the body into front and back. To guide proper body placement you can draw lines on your yoga mat (see figure 3.1). First, to address the sagittal plane, use a ruler to find the middle of your mat, and draw a centerline down the length of the mat. Next, you will establish the top of the mat with a dotted line 8 to 12 inches (20-30 cm) from the top edge. This provides a line to which you always return. There should be enough space

(continued)

to place your hands a few inches in front of your toes when you are standing in a forward fold with your toes touching that line. Once the top of the mat is established, it doesn't change during the standing sequence, just like the centerline. The next sets of lines are represented by the dotted lines, which show the width of your shoulders above the top-of-the-mat line and the width of your hips below the top-of-the-mat line.

We all know our hands are supposed to be shoulder-width apart in the push-up position, and the feet are hip-width apart. Very few people know this actual measurement—they simply guess. We want the placement to be precise, and one way to accomplish this is to mark these widths on the mat. Lie on your back on your mat and have a friend measure the distance between your shoulders and between your hips. Mark those points on your mat. If you don't have someone to help you, you can also use a measuring tape to measure your shoulder and hip widths, then apply those measurements to your mat. Note: When measuring your shoulders, measure from the bony protrusion on top of your shoulder, not the outside of your shoulder. You want to get as close to the shoulder joint as possible, not measuring the extra flesh and muscles on the upper arm. Similarly, for the hips, try to measure from the bony points in front of the hips, not the width of the outer hips.

Create these lines to fit your mat to your body and to guide alignment that will allow you to make sense of the choices you have when practicing standing asanas and to build a proper foundation (hands and feet) for the pose. Use a ruler, and keep your lines straight. Be creative and give yourself something pleasing and easy to observe when practicing. Put lines on your favorite yoga towel if you practice with a towel instead of directly on the mat.

Today, many yoga mats come with lines already marked. Although these are useful for finding the centerline, you may still need to add your specific shoulder-width and hip-width measurements. Over time, your body will be able to feel your foundation and know when it is aligned without the use of lines on your mat.

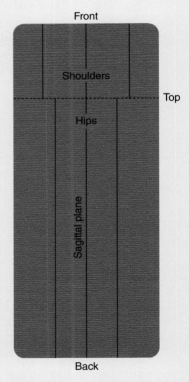

Figure 3.1 Yoga mat lines to guide proper alignment.

Tempo

The progressive ashtanga vinyasa system modifies the postures to provide more accessibility to each student. Progressive ashtanga vinyasa also modifies the tempo of the breath to enhance the overall effects of the practice. For beginners, it is useful to apply a slower breathing tempo to allow for explanation of alignment techniques and to provide an easy environment for learning the postures. This also encourages the mind to slow down and become more aware of the yoga process and its communication with the body.

Rocket yoga's more advanced sequences speed the rhythm to a three- to five-second count for inhalation and exhalation. This juices up the body's fluids and heightens the senses for an empowering practice. The depth of the breath should never be shortened while tempo is changed. The deeper the breath, the deeper the practice will become. Encourage the breath to be profound and deep so that increasing the rhythm does not feel rushed.

TIPS FOR TEACHERS

Setting the Tempo

Knowing how to set the right tempo for your class will come with time. It is important to intuit how your students feel and counteract that to help them achieve balance. If they are stressed from work and moving quickly, slow them with your rhythm to bring them into the present moment. If they seem sluggish or low in energy, increasing your tempo will help to move them into a state of balance and presence.

The timbre and cadence of your voice as well as the cues you provide will stimulate your students through slower or faster tempos. Speaking loudly and quickly will invigorate your students. Alternatively, a quiet and slower cadence will have a calming effect. Record yourself teaching either a full class or just a few rounds of sun salutations. Listen to your voice. Notice the tone of your natural speaking voice. Is it naturally fast and energetic? Is it deep and slow? What small changes can you make to how you speak to affect the tempo of the class?

Music

Sound and music are important considerations in your own personal practice and when creating an experience for your students if you teach. Music can enhance the experience of the practice, but when chosen poorly, it can be distracting. In the classical ashtanga method, no music is used during classes, and the sound of the ujjayi breath becomes the rhythm of the class. The silence creates an atmosphere in which the breath is the primary sound in the practice room, adding to the meditative flow of the practice.

Rocket yoga allows music, which amplifies the energy in the practice, providing yet another outlet of creativity, expression, and expansion. Take a few considerations into account when choosing music for practice. Before you start your practice, decide how you are feeling and what kind of energy you are seeking to cultivate. The music you choose can set the energy and atmosphere for your practice. Don't use music that has a fast rhythm when you want to slow or ease the practice. Also, if you want to invigorate your practice with high energy, slower meditative music will not aid this effect.

Instrumental vs. Lyrics

The easiest music to use for practicing is instrumentals that carry the particular rhythm or tempo that you want to feel. Instrumentals are less distracting than music with lyrics. Words and language ignite a specific part of the brain, and using music with words can be distracting.

Yoga Music vs. Mainstream Music

Students and teachers have different tastes in the type of music that inspires them. Whether you lean toward music created specifically for yoga, like ancient chanting (mantras) or classical ragas, or have a more modern and mainstream music taste inspired by electronic dance music (EDM), there is music for everyone. What is important is that you choose music that is authentic to you, music that you truly enjoy listening and moving to.

Synchronizing Music to Movement

The tempo of the music should match or encourage the same energy being cultivated through movement. The sun salutations and beginning of the standing asanas should have an upbeat rhythm that builds and keeps the tempo of the practice steady. As the forward folds in the standing series are entered, the music tempo slows and coincides with the milder energy of forward folding. With the seated series, there can again be a buildup in the rhythm to keep the mind and body active and engaged. Finishing-series music should slow and encourage introspection. These suggestions on how to work with music apply to all three Rocket yoga sequences.

Silence

It can be useful to work with silence in yoga practice because it focuses the attention on the sound of the breath. It is important to leave a space for silence at the beginning of practice before chanting *om* or during savasana at the end of the practice. If you use music during savasana, it should be light with no loud or sudden sounds.

Additionally, at any moment during practice, the music can be silenced to bring more attention to the sound of the breath. Silence is important because it allows the senses to turn inward, bringing observation within the body.

Choosing Music

Choose music that allows your voice to become the song or lyric that matches the beat as it guides the body through the practice like a dance. If you choose songs that have lyrics, make sure that you understand the lyrics, that they are not offensive, and that they do not contradict the vibe of your class. Positive lyrics and melodic voice tones can sometimes be a positive addition to your class.

Create a 60- to 90-minute playlist, using the guide here:

- *Opening*: a few minutes to set the tone for the practice and begin the sun salutations (5-10 minutes)
- *Warming up*: moving into the standing sequence (10-15 minutes)
- *Peak movement*: the most physically intense portion of the practice (20-25 minutes)
- *Cooling down*: bringing the energy of the practice back down with slower movements or longer holds in poses (10-15 minutes)
- *Finishing*: finishing sequence and final poses (10-15 minutes)
- *Savasana*: allowing rest, with music or in silence (5-10 minutes)

Sequence

Rocket yoga is simply a reconfiguration of the sequence of traditional poses. Studying the subsequences of each routine will help you to understand the overall sequence of the entire practice. The subsequences are the smaller chunks within the series that have a common theme. Every practice begins with sun salutations A and B, followed by a sequence of standing poses known as the standing sequence. This is followed by a set of seated poses from either the classical ashtanga primary or intermediate series. All practices end with the same sequence targeted at cooling the body, known as the finishing sequence. You will notice similarities and overlap between the sequences of classical ashtanga and Rocket yoga, but starting with sun salutations and the standing sequence and ending with the finishing sequence is always the same.

The base sequences of Rocket yoga do not add extra or new poses to the standing sequence. You should be familiar with the traditional series first and then progress into the deeper science of sequencing with the Rocket routines. Learn the variations as smaller sequences that can be added on to help encourage specific effects in the practice. Nothing is better than practice. Teachers ideally practice the same sequence they teach each day or a more advanced variation of that sequence.

TIPS FOR TEACHERS

Expanding Your Vocabulary

As a teacher, the words you use have an impact not only on the tone of the class but also on the experience the student has. Expanding your vocabulary can help you to be more specific in the experience that you build. Applying stimulating vocabulary encourages depth and creativity for both you and your students. In addition, knowing how to express an idea in multiple ways creates efficient communication between what you would like your students to do or feel and what they actually do and feel.

Here is a list of words you can start to weave into your classes. Write down any words from other teachers that resonate with you. Write your own list of words that feel authentic to you and that you would like to remember for future classes.

Adjectives and Adverbs	Verbs	
Aware	Affirm	Lengthen
Beautiful	Anchor	Melt
Compassionate	Articulate	Pause
Conscious	Ascend	Peel
Crystal clear	Assimilate	Play
Deep	Center	Pour
Direct	Contemplate	Probe
Divine	Create	Reach
Electric	Descend	Refresh
Elegant	Embody	Release
Energetic	Empower	Retreat
Expansive	Engage	Ride
Expressive	Enlighten	Salute
Freeing	Enliven	Sip
Fresh	Explore	Stimulate
Grounded	Extend	Support
Light	Exude	Surrender
Luscious	Flex	Synchronize
Melting	Flow	Transcend
Molding	Glide	Transform
Rooted	Ground	Validate
Spacious	Grow	Wiggle
Truthful	Integrate	Wander
		Wonder

*Firmness,
or Yang Energy*

Aspire
Bold
Confidence
Courage
Dynamic
Energetic
Equilibrium
Faith
Fearlessness
Focused
Fortitude
Independence
Inner flowing
Integrity
Intention
Patience
Purity

Rational
Resolute
Resolution
Humility
Steadfast
Stillness
Tolerance
Trust
Truthfulness
Vigor
Vitality
Willpower

Yin Energy

Allow
Celebrate
Connect
Compassion
Devotional
Enthusiasm

Feminine
Generosity
Gentle
Gratitude
Happiness
Intuitive
Kindness
Love
Mindfulness
Open
Opening
Passive
Receptive
Reverent
Soft
Subtle
Surrender
Wise
Yielding

Incorporating Creativity

The classical ashtanga sequences as well as the foundational Rocket sequences are meant to guide your practice and provide a road map that relies on the power of repetition to boost your practice. By practicing the same set of sequences, you will notice the physical changes in your body, and your mind will begin to relax, confident in the sequence of poses.

Now is the time to listen to your body and to the manifestations of creativity that begin to emerge. If you find yourself wanting to experiment with the different physical forms, feel free to do so. Trying different variations, spending more time on a pose, or adding drills will empower your practice. Your body has its own intuition, and the beauty of Rocket yoga lies in its flexibility that allows each yogi to work where they are most comfortable at that very moment. In chapter 10, we will cover ways you can modify this practice to suit where you are at a specific time.

Keep in mind that the feeling of being inside the pose is important. This feeling, which is an ideal balance between stimulation and comfort, guides you to the shape inside the pose that is best for your body. Therefore, modifications to make the practice more accessible for stiffer or less conditioned bodies and variations to make the practice more stimulating and challenging will be the result of exploration and creativity in your practice. Creativity might be something as subtle as experimenting with your hand position (open hand versus closed fist) or where your eyes are looking. It can also be something more dramatic such as lifting a foot off the floor to turn a standing posture into a balancing posture or adding a twist where there usually isn't one.

Creativity drives the evolution of personal process. Learning to listen to your inner teacher will open new experiences in your body's capabilities with movement and in your mind's capabilities with perception.

TIPS FOR TEACHERS

Theming a Class

When looking to bring new techniques or postures into your classes, it is helpful to work around a theme or specific intention. This can be subtle, such as emphasizing ahimsa throughout the practice, or it can be more direct and physical, such as opening the hips or strengthening the upper body. The subtle effects of weaving a theme through a class help to draw students deeper into the feeling of the practice and self-observation.

These themes can show themselves throughout the sequence, with more detail brought to preparatory postures or through building up the core concepts of new postures. Repetition is key for the process of the body's learning. Themes should carry themselves throughout a weekly or even monthly process for students to fully integrate the new postures and the lessons of the theme. It is useful to convey the theme of the class to the students so that they can join in the process of bringing attention and detail to different areas of the body.

As an exercise, write a theme for a class. How can you relate this theme to the basic fundamental postures in Rocket yoga? What postures can you integrate or emphasize to iterate your theme? What cues can you provide to bring the student's awareness to the theme and how it correlates to their practice?

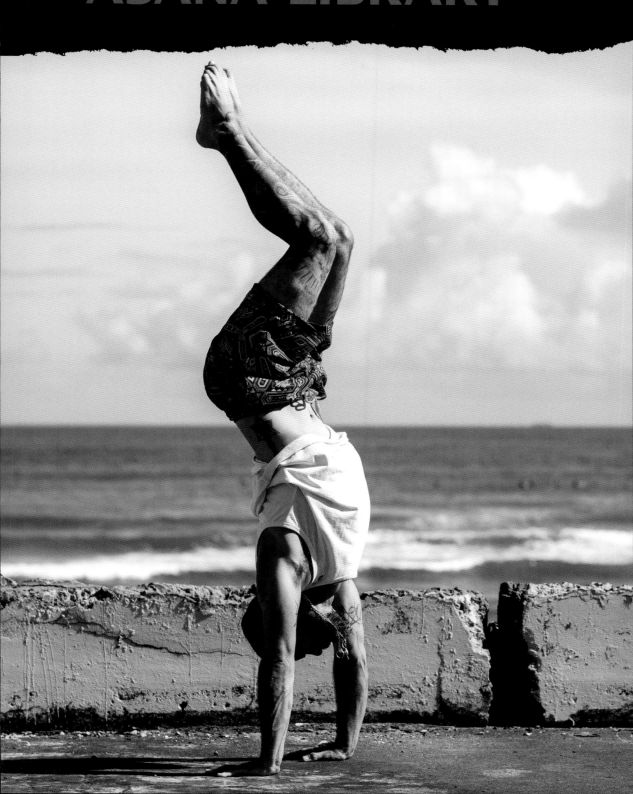

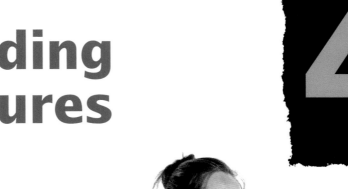

Standing Postures

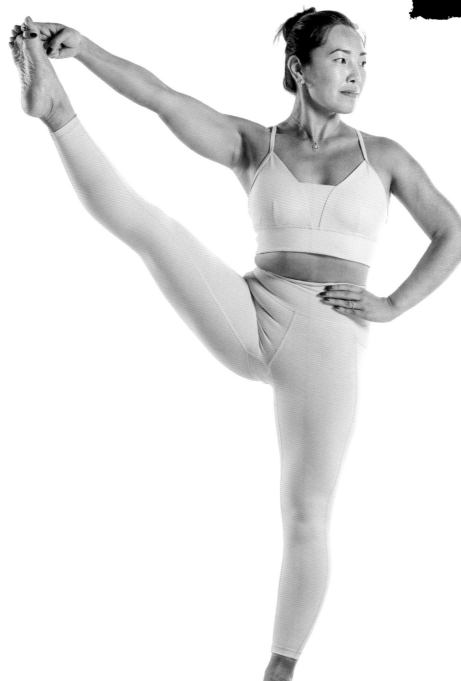

The standing postures are performed at the beginning of both the classical ashtanga and Rocket yoga series, albeit with some variation. They warm up the legs and create a grounding energy from which the rest of the practice can unfold.

All of the standing poses in Rocket yoga come from classical ashtanga. The notable difference is the sequence that they are practiced in and the addition of arm balances and inversions that amplify the grounding energy. As you practice both sequences, notice which one feels better in your body. Do you feel more physically warmed up with one sequence? Do you feel a greater grounding energy with the other? Tap into this self-exploration to guide your practice.

SAMASTHITI

(sahm-as-TEE-tee)

sama = equal, same   sthiti = standing pose

EQUAL STANDING POSE

First drishti: nasikagra—tip of the nose

1. Stand on the mat with the feet together. Arms are relaxed at the side of the body. Head is neutral. Evenly distribute weight on all four corners of the feet.
2. Press the base of the big toes into the mat to engage pada bandha.
3. Draw the navel into the spine to engage uddiyana bandha.

Modification

To help with balance, stand with the feet hip-width apart.

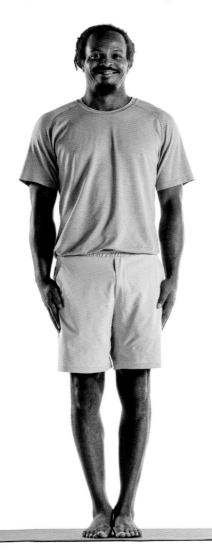

URDHVA HASTASANA
(OORD-vah ahs-TAS-ahna)

urdhva = upward   hasta = hands   asana = pose

UPWARD SALUTE

Eighth drishti: angustha ma dyai—thumb

1. From samasthiti (page 51), on an inhale, raise the arms above the head, pressing the palms together at the top.
2. Draw the navel into the spine to engage uddiyana bandha.

Modification

To ease shoulder tension, bring hands shoulder-width apart.

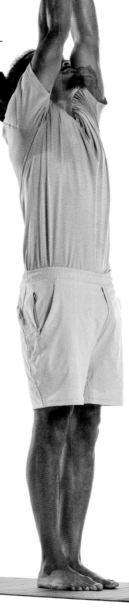

TADASANA VARIATION

(tah-DAHS-anna)

tada = mountain   asana = pose

MOUNTAIN POSE (WITH HEELS LIFTED)

First drishti: nasikagra—tip of the nose

1. From uttanasana variation (page 71), on an inhale, straighten the legs and roll up the spine one vertebra at a time until fully erect. Raise both hands overhead, turning the palms toward the centerline and keeping them shoulder-width apart.

2. On an exhale, lift the heels, balancing on the balls of the feet. Stretch the body completely from the toes to the fingertips. Pull the front ribs into the body to prevent the back from arching. Aim to create a hollow front body, feeling the pose as a handstand on the feet. Press evenly into the balls of the feet to avoid balancing on the inner or outer edge of the foot.

3. Scoop the sacrum under and draw the navel into the spine to engage uddiyana bandha and stabilize the core. Engage the inner thighs toward the midline to lift the pelvic floor and engage mula bandha. Maintain the soft sound of the breath through the contraction of the throat to gently apply jalandhara bandha.

4. After a few breaths, walk forward on the balls of the feet to return to the top of the mat for samasthiti.

Modification

To aid with balance, leave the heels down, and focus on lengthening the spine.

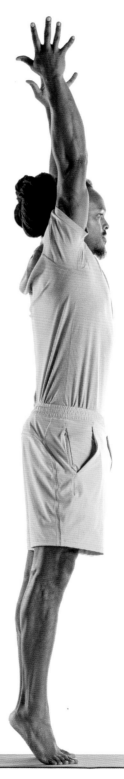

CHATURANGA DANDASANA

(CHAT-oor-an-gah dahn-DAS-ahna)

catur = four   anga = limb   danda = staff   asana = pose

FOUR-LIMBED STAFF POSE
LOW PLANK

First drishti: nasikagra—tip of the nose

1. From uttanasana (page 70), place the palms flat on the ground shoulder-width apart.
2. Step the feet back so the body is in a high plank, forming one line from the shoulders to the heels.
3. Bend the elbows, and lower the body until the elbows are at 90 degrees and pointing toward the back of the mat. Keep the entire body as straight as possible during the motion.
4. Draw the navel into the spine to engage uddiyana bandha.

Modification

If you do not have the strength to perform the full chaturanga from high plank, lower the knees to the ground, and from this position, bend the elbows to lower to the ground.

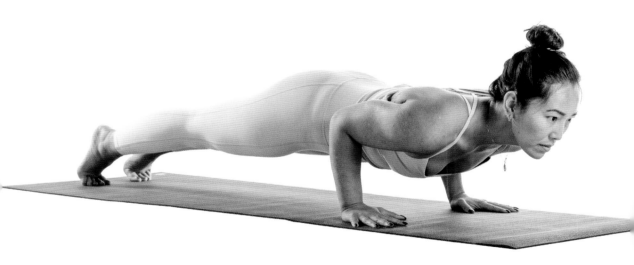

URDHVA MUKHA SVANASANA

(OORD-vah MOO-kah shvah-NAHS-ahna)

urdhva = upward   mukha = facing   svana = dog   asana = pose

UPWARD-FACING DOG

First drishti: nasikagra—tip of the nose

1. From chaturanga dandasana (page 54), straighten the arms completely, keeping the hips and lower body close to the ground.
2. Untuck the toes so the tops of the toes touch the mat.
3. Engage the quads and lift the knees off the ground.
4. Draw the torso and ribs through the arms, keeping the shoulders away from the ears. Lift the chin slightly.
5. Draw the navel into the spine to engage uddiyana bandha.

Modification

Keeping the knees on the ground, straighten the arms only halfway and lift the head and collarbones using the upper-back muscles.

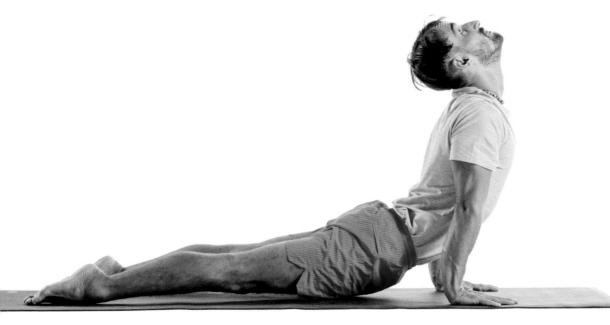

ADHO MUKHA SVANASANA

(AH-doh MOO-kah shvah-NAHS-ahna)

adho = downward   mukha = facing   svana = dog   asana = pose

DOWNWARD-FACING DOG

Third drishti: nabhi chakra—navel

1. From urdhva mukha svanasana (page 55), on an exhale, keep the hands and feet in place as you lift the hips to form an inverted V shape.
2. Press the thighs toward the back of the mat, and then press into the hands to move the rib cage toward the thighs.
3. Lower the heels toward the ground as much as possible.
4. Draw the navel into the spine to engage uddiyana bandha.

Modification

To ease the hamstring stretch, bend the knees generously.

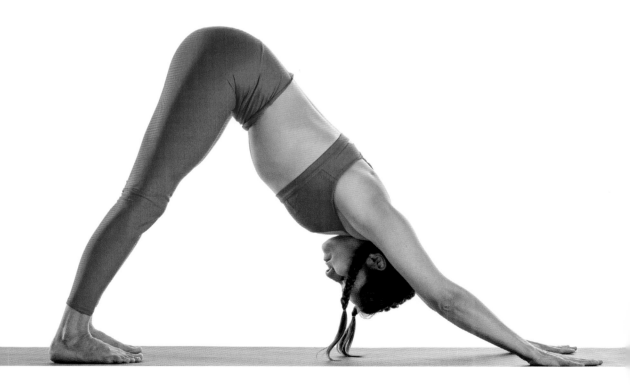

UTKATASANA
(OOT-kah-TAHS-anna)
utkata = fierce, powerful   asana = pose

FIERCE POSE

CHAIR POSE

AWKWARD POSTURE

Eighth drishti: angustha ma dyai—thumb

1. From samasthiti (page 51), on an inhale, bend the knees as much as possible while keeping the heels on the ground and the torso erect. Raise both arms overhead, press the palms together, and reach the fingers toward the sky.

2. Keep the big toes, ankles, and knees touching by engaging the inner thighs. Keep the weight on the feet evenly distributed between the ball of the foot and heels. Tuck the tailbone, aligning the tops of hip bones parallel to the floor. Lift the sternum to open the heart, and pull the front ribs in to secure the front of the body.

3. Draw the navel into the spine to engage uddiyana bandha. Lift the pelvic floor to engage mula bandha. Maintain the soft sound of the breath through the contraction of the throat to gently apply jalandhara bandha.

Modifications

- To ease shoulder tension, bring the hands shoulder-width apart.
- To reduce work in the legs, decrease the bend in the knees.
- To aid with balance, widen the stance side to side.
- To ease neck tension, shift the drishti forward to lengthen the back of the neck.

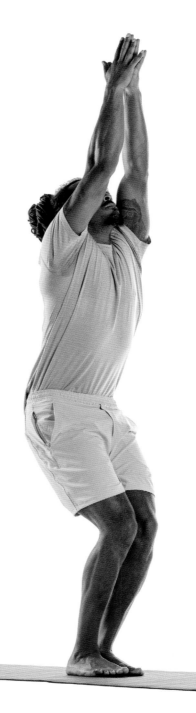

ARDHA UTKATASANA
(ARD-hah OOT-kah-TAHS-anna)

ardha = half   utkata = fierce, powerful   asana = pose

HALF-CHAIR POSE

First drishti: nasikagra—tip of the nose

1. From utkatasana (page 57), on an exhale, bring the torso parallel to the floor until it is just touching the upper thigh. Both the thighs and the torso are parallel to the ground. Clasp the hands and raise the arms above the ears to prevent the upper back from rounding forward.

2. Reach the crown of the head forward and the tailbone back in opposition to lengthen the spine. Keep the weight of the body shifted back into the heels to prevent them from lifting. This will engage the thighs more.

3. Draw the navel into the spine to lift the belly off the thighs and engage uddiyana bandha. Press the heels down, squeeze the inner thighs together, and lift the pelvic floor to engage mula bandha. Maintain the soft sound of the breath through the contraction of the throat to gently apply jalandhara bandha.

Modifications

- To ease shoulder tension, bring the hands shoulder-width apart.
- To reduce work in the legs, decrease the bend in the knees.
- To aid with balance, widen the stance side to side.

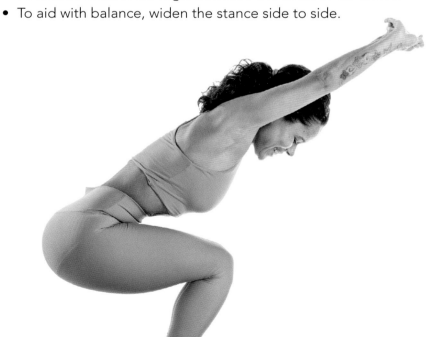

KAKASANA

(kah-KAHS-ahna)

kaka = crow   asana = pose

CROW POSE

First drishti: nasikagra—tip of the nose

1. From utkatasana (page 57), place both palms on the floor, shoulder-width apart. Bring the knees either to the top of the elbow, to the top of the triceps, or to the outside of the triceps. Look forward and lean forward to bring the weight of the body to the hands.
2. Lift both feet off the ground. Engage the inner thighs to keep the big toes touching.
3. Continue to push both hands into the ground and balance on the hands.
4. Lift the pelvic floor to engage mula bandha and draw the navel into the spine to engage uddiyana bandha.

Modifications

- To relieve weight on the wrists, lift only the heels from the mat until the wrists are strong enough to support the body weight.
- To work on balance, lift one foot at a time, alternating between feet.

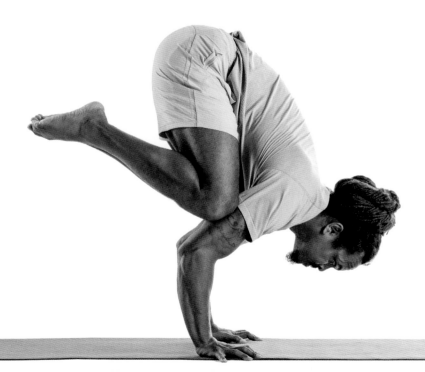

BAKASANA A

(bahk-AHS-anna)

baka = crane   asana = pose

CRANE POSE

First drishti: nasikagra—tip of the nose

1. From ardha utkatasana (page 58), on an exhale, place the hands on the mat shoulder-width apart, spreading the fingers to broaden the surface space and stabilize the wrists.
2. Bend the elbows, placing the knees on the shelf created by the upper arms. Place the knees as close as possible to the armpits. Shift the weight forward from the feet to the hands, and lift the feet by engaging the hamstrings.
3. Move the elbows forward until they stack over the wrists. Move the weight on the hands to the balls of the hands and fingers. This will allow you to use the entire hand to help with balance. Squeeze the inner thighs toward the midline for more lift.
4. On an exhale, straighten the arms. Press the knees firmly into the arms, and pull the thighs into the chest.
5. Draw the navel into the spine to engage uddiyana bandha. Lift the pelvic floor to engage mula bandha.

Modifications

- To relieve weight on the wrists, lift only the heels from the mat until the wrists are strong enough to support the body weight.
- To work on balance, lift one foot at a time, alternating feet.
- A block can be used to support the feet in an upright position, simulating the feeling of balance in the full pose.

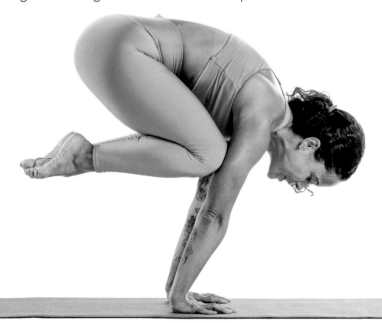

VIRABHADRASANA A

(veer-ah-bah-DRAHS-anna)

virabhadra = warrior   asana = pose

WARRIOR I

Fourth drishti: hastagrai—hand or fingertips

1. From adho mukha svanasana (page 56), on an inhale, step one foot forward into a lunge, rotating the back heel in 45 degrees to press the heel and the outer edge of the back foot into the floor.

2. Raise both arms overhead, clasp the hands together and interlace the fingers, and then press the palms toward the sky.

3. As much as possible, keep the ribs and hips square to the front of the mat. Bring the forward knee over the ankle to create a 90-degree angle, allowing the thigh of the forward leg to lower until it is parallel to the ground.

4. Without moving either foot, engage the inner thighs as though bringing the legs together in the center. This will create an opposition that strengthens the legs.

5. Draw the navel into the spine to engage uddiyana bandha, and keep the breath in the heart space. Lift the pelvic floor to engage mula bandha. Maintain the soft sound of the breath through the contraction of the throat to gently apply jalandhara bandha.

6. Repeat on the other side.

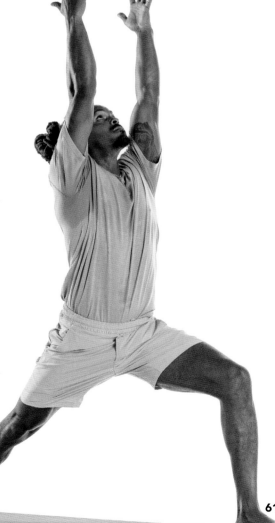

Modifications

- To ease shoulder tension, bring the hands shoulder-width apart.

- To aid with balance, widen the stance side to side.

- To ease the opening of the hips, lift the back heel, shorten the stance, or decrease the angle of the lunge.

VIRABHADRASANA B

(veer-ah-bah-DRAHS-anna)

virabhadra = warrior   asana = pose

WARRIOR II

Fourth drishti: hastagrai—hand or fingertips

1. From virabhadrasana A (page 61), on an exhale, open the hips toward the side of the mat and allow the feet to slide a little farther apart. Release the clasp of the hands, and open the arms to the sides until they are parallel to the floor and aligned over the legs.

2. Bring the forward knee over the ankle to create a 90-degree angle, allowing the thigh of the forward leg to lower until it is parallel to the ground. Without moving either foot, engage the inner thighs as though bringing the legs together in the center. This will create an opposition that strengthens the legs. Press the heel and the outer edge of the back foot into the floor, maintaining a lifted arch in the back foot.

3. Gently tuck the tailbone to balance the pelvis, keeping the spine perpendicular to the ground. Draw the shoulder blades down the back to lift the chest.

4. Draw the navel into the spine to engage uddiyana bandha and keep the breath in the heart space. Lift the pelvic floor to engage mula bandha. Maintain the soft sound of the breath through the contraction of the throat to gently apply jalandhara bandha.

5. Repeat on the other side.

Modifications

- To ease shoulder tension, turn the palms toward the sky.
- To aid with balance, widen the stance side to side.
- To ease the opening of the hips, turn the back foot out to 90 degrees, shorten the stance, or decrease the angle of the lunge.

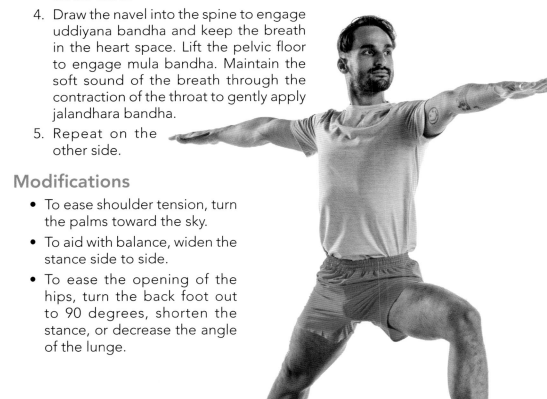

UTTHITA TRIKONASANA

(oo-TEE-tah tree-cohn-AHS-anna)

utthita = extended   tri = three   kona = angle   asana = pose

TRIANGLE POSE

Eighth drishti: angustha ma dyai—thumb

1. From virabhadrasana B (page 62), on an inhale, straighten the front leg, keeping the arms in the T position out to the sides.
2. On an exhale, extend the torso over the forward leg. Reach the bottom hand toward the forward foot. With the first two fingers, clasp the big toe of the forward foot while reaching up with the upper arm, creating opposition that opens across the heart space.
3. Avoid collapsing the torso by opening the chest toward the sky. Avoid overextension of the spine by gently tucking the tailbone. Move the lower hip under as the upper hip opens to align the hips.
4. Draw the navel into the spine to engage uddiyana bandha and keep the breath in the heart space. Lift the pelvic floor to engage mula bandha. Maintain the soft sound of the breath through the contraction of the throat to gently apply jalandhara bandha.
5. Repeat on the other side.

Modifications

- To decrease the stretch on the hamstring or the side body or both, place the lower hand onto a block, the ankle, or the shin.
- To align the upper body with the legs, set up the pose with your back to a wall, then lean back into the wall as you move into the pose.

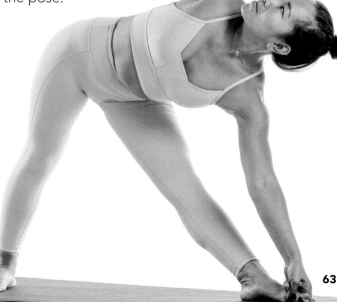

PARIVRTTA TRIKONASANA

(par-ee-VREET-tah tree-cohn-AHS-anna)

parivrtta = revolved   tri = three   kona = angle   asana = pose

REVOLVED TRIANGLE POSE

Eighth drishti: angustha ma dyai—thumb

1. From utthita trikonasana (page 63), on an exhale, look down toward the ground, and then step the back foot in to shorten the stance enough to square the hips to the front of the mat.

2. On an inhale, bring the opposite hand to the outside of the forward foot, pressing the palm into the ground. Reach the other hand toward the sky. Lengthen and twist from the base of the spine, opening the chest toward the sky.

3. Keep the hips square to stabilize the base of the spine, lengthening through the crown of the head and extending back through the sacrum.

4. Push down into the ground with the bottom hand to provide the rotation and twist needed for the top hand to reach higher. Distribute the weight evenly between the legs to stabilize the pelvis further.

5. Draw the navel into the spine to engage uddiyana bandha and keep the breath in the heart space. Engage the inner thighs toward the midline to lift the pelvic floor and engage mula bandha. Bring the chin toward the shoulder to gently apply jalandhara bandha.

6. Repeat on the other side.

Modifications

- To aid with balance, widen the stance side to side.

- To decrease the stretch on the hamstrings or side body or both, place the lower hand onto a block, the ankle, or the shin.

- To decrease the tension induced by twisting the spine, place both hands on the floor or on blocks to emphasize the work in the legs.

- To secure the base of the spine for twisting, place the top hand on the sacrum, focusing on keeping it square to the ground during the twisting motion.

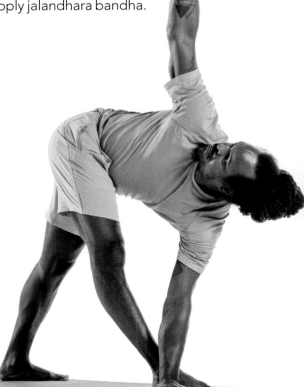

UTTHITA PARSVAKONASANA

(oo-TEE-tah pars-vah-cohn-AHS-anna)

utthita = extended   parsva = side   kona = angle   asana = pose

EXTENDED SIDE ANGLE POSE

Fourth drishti: hastagrai—hand or fingertips

1. From parivrtta trikonasana (page 64), on an exhale, look toward the ground. Use both hands to bend the front knee, and step the back foot farther back to take a wider stance, allowing the hips to open to the side of the mat. The front thigh creates a 90-degree angle to the shin. The shoulders are in line with the hips. The forward hand is placed with the palm flat on the ground outside of the forward foot.

2. On an inhale, reach the back arm above the head and forward at a 45-degree angle, creating a long line along the side of the body from the outer edge of the back foot to the hand of the top arm. Spin the chest up toward the sky.

3. Press the outside of the front knee into the arm that is pressing into the ground. This action will open the inner thigh and pelvis. If the front knee moves past a 90-degree angle, slide the back foot farther to lengthen the stance.

4. Draw the navel into the spine to engage uddiyana bandha and keep the breath in the heart space. Engage the inner thighs toward the midline to lift the pelvic floor and engage mula bandha. Bring the chin toward the shoulder to gently apply jalandhara bandha.

5. Repeat on the other side.

Modifications

- To decrease compression in the hip, do not place the forward hand on the floor. Instead, bring the elbow to the top of the thigh, creating more space in the hip and side body.

- To focus more on the alignment of the torso, reach the top arm straight up to the sky.

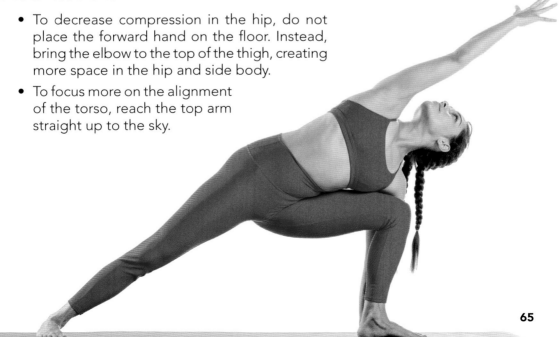

PARIVRTTA PARSVAKONASANA

(par-ee-VREET-tah pars-vah-cohn-AHS-anna)

parivrtta = revolved   parsva = side   kona = angle   asana = pose

REVOLVED SIDE ANGLE POSE

Fourth drishti: hastagrai–hand or fingertips

1. From utthita parsvakonasana (page 65), on an inhale, return to standing and square the torso and hips to the front of the mat, keeping the deep bend in the front knee.

2. On an exhale, twist from the base of the spine toward the front knee, placing the opposite elbow outside of the knee. Extend the arm so the hand reaches to the ground outside of the foot, pressing the palm firmly into the ground. Extend the other arm over the head to create a straight line from the outer edge of the back foot through the middle finger of the top hand.

3. Apply extra effort into maintaining deep breaths in twisting postures that apply more compression to the torso. The downward pressure in the bottom hand is essential for opening the twist of the spine, even if just the fingertips keep reaching into the ground as the chest rotates and opens toward the sky.

4. Keep downward pressure on both feet by engaging the inner thighs toward the midline to lift the pelvic floor and engage mula bandha. Draw the navel into the spine to engage uddiyana bandha, lifting the belly to provide space for more rotation of the spine. Bring the chin toward the shoulder to gently apply jalandhara bandha.

5. Repeat on the other side.

Modifications

- To emphasize the rotation of the spine, when bringing the outside of the elbow to the opposite knee, press the palms together in prayer, and bring the thumbs to the center of the sternum.

- To ease the opening of the hips, shorten the stance and decrease the angle of the lunge.

- To aid with balance, lift the back heel or completely drop the back knee to the ground.

PINCHA MAYURASANA

(PEEN-cha my-oor-AHS-anna)

pincha = feather   mayura = peacock   asana = pose

LIFTED PEACOCK FEATHER POSE

FOREARM STAND

First drishti: nasikagra—tip of the nose

1. From adho mukha svanasana (page 56), on an exhale, drop the knees and elbows to the ground to prepare. Grab opposite elbows to measure a forearm's length between the elbows, then straighten the forearms so they are parallel with the sides of the mat. Spread the fingers wide, rotate the upper arms externally, and press the forearms firmly into the mat.

2. Lift the knees off the mat, and walk the feet in toward the elbows, beginning to shift weight from the legs to the arms.

3. On an inhale, gently kick up with one or two legs until both legs are extended straight over the hips and shoulders. Squeeze the elbows toward one another to stabilize the foundation. Keep the body active and firm for easier balance.

4. Engage the bandhas by tucking the tailbone for uddiyana bandha, and squeeze the legs together to awaken mula bandha. Press into the shoulder blades to lengthen the neck and prevent the shoulders from collapsing.

5. Hold for as long as needed.

6. On an exhale, lower the legs to the mat with control, straighten the elbows, and press into downward-facing dog.

Modifications

- If maintaining a parallel position in the forearms is difficult, change the foundation of your forearms by placing one hand on top of the other to create a triangular foundation.

- If there is not sufficient strength to carry the weight of the body in the shoulders, lift only one leg toward the sky for dolphin pose. Practice both sides.

- Practice the forearm plank position for shoulder stabilization without the balance.

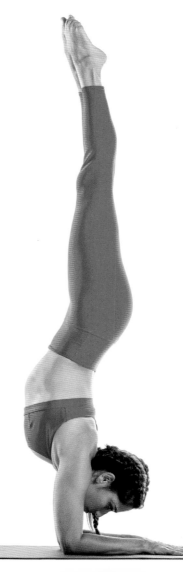

67

PADANGUSTHASANA

(pod-ang-goosh-TAHS-anna)

pada = foot   angustha = big toe   asana = pose

BIG TOE POSE

Third drishti: nabhi chakra—navel

1. From adho mukha svanasana (page 56), walk the hands toward the back of the mat, coming into a forward-folding position with the feet hip-width apart and parallel. Clasp the big toes with the first two fingers of both hands.
2. On an inhale, look up, lift the chest, and pull the shoulder blades back and down.
3. On an exhale, lengthen the spine and fold forward, allowing the elbows to extend out toward the sides while the crown of the head reaches toward the floor. Shoulders lift away from the ears to relax the shoulders. Engage the front of the thighs to release tension in the hamstrings. Allow the crown of the head to reach slightly forward and down to prevent the spine from rounding excessively.
4. Draw the navel into the spine to engage uddiyana bandha even before bending forward and keep the breath in the heart space. Engage the inner thighs toward the midline to lift the pelvic floor and engage mula bandha. Maintain the soft sound of the breath through the contraction of the throat to gently apply jalandhara bandha.

Modification

To ease the hamstring stretch, bend the knees generously.

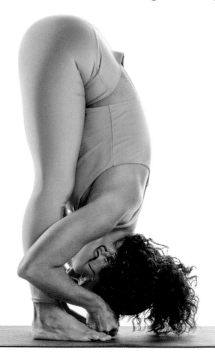

PADAHASTASANA
(pah-dah-has-TAHS-anna)

pada = foot   hasta = hand   asana = pose

FOOT TO HAND POSE

Third drishti: nabhi chakra—navel

1. From padangusthasana (page 68), on an inhale, look up and lift the torso to extend the spine. Release the big toes, then slide the palms under the soles of the feet with palms facing upward until the toes come all the way to the wrist creases.

2. On an exhale, fold forward, maintaining the length in the spine. Allow the elbows to bend out toward the side or back toward the body. Balance the weight in the feet evenly from the balls of the feet to the heels. Shoulders lift away from the ears to relax shoulders. Engage the front of the thighs to release tension in the hamstrings. Allow the crown of the head to reach slightly forward and down to prevent the spine from rounding excessively.

3. Draw the navel into the spine to engage uddiyana bandha even before bending forward and keep the breath in the heart space. Engage the inner thighs toward the midline to lift the pelvic floor and engage mula bandha. Maintain the soft sound of the breath through the contraction of the throat to gently apply jalandhara bandha.

Modification

To ease the hamstring stretch, bend the knees generously.

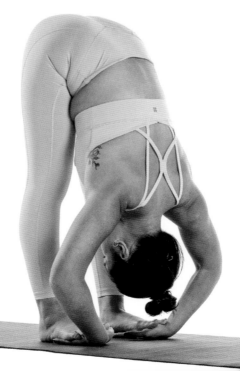

UTTANASANA

(OOT-tan-AHS-ahna)

ut = intense, powerful, deliberate
tan = stretch, lengthen   asana = pose

INTENSE STRETCH

STANDING FORWARD FOLD

Third drishti: nabhi chakra—navel

1. From samasthiti (page 51), fold forward, hinging from the hips.
2. Draw the navel into the spine to engage uddiyana bandha.

Modification

To ease the hamstring stretch and lower-back stretch, bend the knees generously, resting the front of the ribs on top of the thighs.

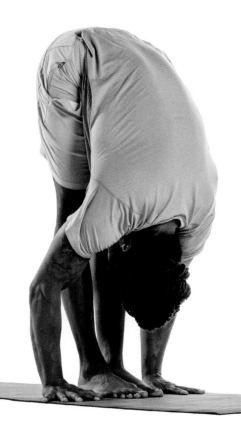

UTTANASANA VARIATION

(OOT-tan-AHS-ahna)

ut = intense   tan = stretch   asana = pose

INTENSE STRETCH

Third drishti: nabhi chakra—navel

1. From padahastasana (page 69), on an inhale, look up and lift the torso to extend the spine and stretch the back of the wrists.

2. On an exhale, release both hands from under the feet and grab opposite elbows. Relax the torso and allow gravity to pull on the upper body, reaching the elbows toward the tops of the feet. Gently shake the head to release tension in the neck.

3. Draw the navel into the spine to engage uddiyana bandha even before bending forward and keep the breath in the heart space. Engage the inner thighs toward the midline to lift the pelvic floor and engage mula bandha. Maintain the soft sound of the breath through the contraction of the throat to gently apply jalandhara bandha.

Modification

To ease the hamstring stretch, bend the knees generously.

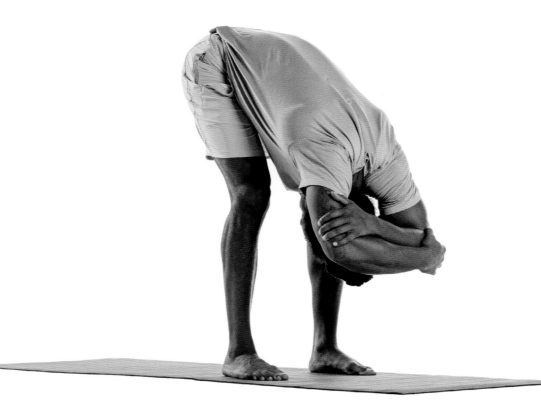

ARDHA UTTANASANA

(AR-dha OOT-tan-AHS-ahna)

ardha = half   ut = intense   tan = stretch   asana = pose

HALF INTENSE STRETCH

HALF LIFT

First drishti: nasikagra—tip of the nose

1. From uttanasana (page 70), keep the hands on the ground, and lift the torso until the arms are straight and the spine is lengthened forward.
2. Draw the navel into the spine to engage uddiyana bandha.

Modification

Place the hands on the front of the shins or the knees and lift the torso halfway from that point, keeping the knees generously bent.

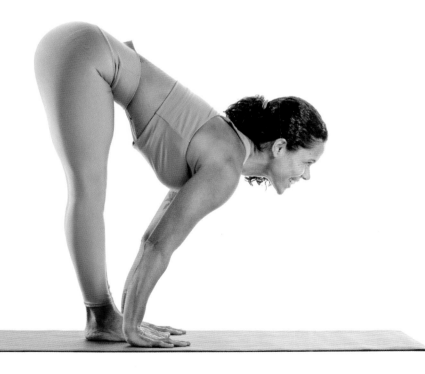

PRASARITA PADOTTANASANA A

(pra-sa-REE-tah pah-doh-tahn-AHS-anna)

prasarita = spread   pada = foot
ut = intense   tan = stretch   asana = pose

WIDE-LEG INTENSE STRETCHING POSE

First drishti: nasikagra—tip of the nose

1. From samasthiti (page 51), on an inhale, step the right foot toward the back of the mat, turn the body to face the side of the mat, and bring the arms out to form a T. The outer edges of the feet are parallel, and the feet are wider than shoulder width. With the arms extended to the side, the feet should be under the forearms, anywhere from under the elbows to under the wrists. When you fold forward, the crown of the head should touch the ground between the feet. Adjust the width of the stance accordingly. Once you find your stance, press the outside edges of the feet into the mat to lift the inner arches of the feet.

2. On an exhale, bring the hands to the waist.

3. On an inhale, reach both arms overhead, and then on an exhale, lengthen the spine and fold forward, placing the hands on the mat shoulder-width apart with the fingertips in line with the toes.

4. On an inhale, lift the torso halfway to establish a strong and straight spine, and then on an exhale, fold forward, bringing the crown of the head toward the ground. Keep the elbows pointed toward the back and bent to 90 degrees. Draw the scapula up the back and away from the shoulders.

5. Engage the inner thighs toward the midline to lift the pelvic floor and engage mula bandha. Lift the belly to engage uddiyana bandha. This will assist in pelvic tilt and support the lower-lumbar area during the compressive nature of the fold. Keep the chin locked to engage jalandhara bandha. This will aid in blood pressure control because blood moves into the head during standing forward folds.

Modifications

- To ease the hamstring stretch, bend the knees generously.
- Place the forehead or hands on blocks to help maintain spinal extension in the forward fold.

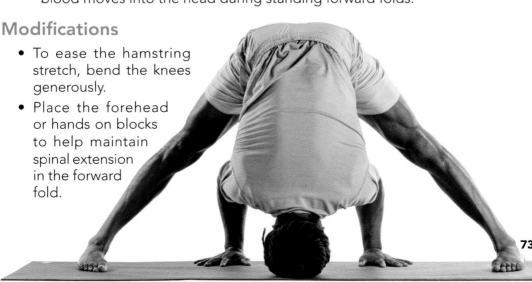

PRASARITA PADOTTANASANA B

(pra-sa-REE-tah pah-doh-tahn-AHS-anna)

prasarita = spread   pada = foot
ut = intense   tan = stretch   asana = pose

WIDE-LEG INTENSE STRETCHING POSE

First drishti: nasikagra—tip of the nose

1. From prasarita padottanasana A (page 73), on an inhale, look up and lift the torso to extend the spine. Stay here for the exhalation, and bring the hands to the waist.
2. On an inhale, stand up all the way and bring the arms over the head, pressing the palms together at the top. Look up toward the thumbs.
3. On an exhale, bring the arms behind the back and place the hands in the reverse prayer position.
4. On an inhale, look up to the sky and press the palms firmly together to open the chest.
5. On an exhale, fold forward at the waist, keeping the elbows open, and place the crown of the head on the floor. Shift the weight forward in the feet so the heels are not heavy and the hips align forward with the legs and feet.
6. Engage the inner thighs toward the midline to lift the pelvic floor and engage mula bandha. Lift the belly to engage uddiyana bandha. This will assist in pelvic tilt and support the lower-lumbar area during the compressive nature of the fold. Keep the chin locked to engage jalandhara bandha. This will aid in blood pressure control because blood moves into the head during standing forward folds.

Modifications

- To ease the hamstring stretch, bend the knees generously.
- Place the forehead or hands on blocks to help to maintain spinal extension in the forward fold.
- To ease shoulder tension, grab opposite elbows or bring the fists together behind the back.

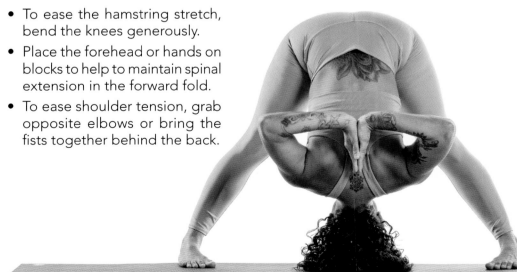

PRASARITA PADOTTANASANA C

(*pra-sa-REE-tah pah-doh-tahn-AHS-anna*)

prasarita = spread   pada = foot
ut = intense   tan = stretch   asana = pose

WIDE-LEG INTENSE STRETCHING POSE

First drishti: nasikagra—tip of the nose

1. From prasarita padottanasana B (page 74), on an inhale, come fully upright, look to the sky, reach the arms overhead, and press the palms firmly together.

2. On an exhale, interlace the fingers behind the back, then straighten the arms to draw the shoulder blades inward and down.

3. On an inhale, look up, open the chest, and extend the crown of the head toward the sky. On an exhale, lift the clasped hands off the back to fold forward, taking care to maintain the neutral spine position. Bring the crown of the head toward the ground.

4. Engage the inner thighs toward the midline to lift the pelvic floor and engage mula bandha. Lift the belly to engage uddiyana bandha. This will assist in pelvic tilt and support the lower lumbar area during the compressive nature of the fold. Keep the chin locked to engage jalandhara bandha. This will aid in blood pressure control because blood moves into the head during standing forward folds.

Modifications

- To ease the hamstring stretch, bend the knees generously.
- Place the forehead or hands on blocks to help to maintain spinal extension in the forward fold. To ease shoulder tension, use a strap to aid with the bind.

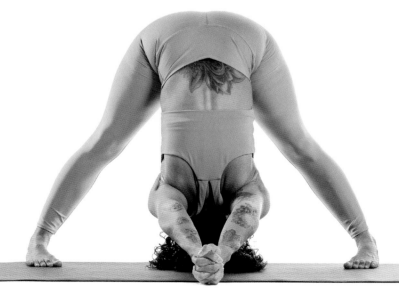

PRASARITA PADOTTANASANA D

(pra-sa-REE-tah pah-doh-tahn-AHS-anna)

prasarita = spread   pada = foot
ut = intense   tan = stretch   asana = pose

WIDE-LEG INTENSE STRETCHING POSE

First drishti: nasikagra—tip of the nose

1. From prasarita padottanasana C (page 75), on an inhale, come fully upright, look to the sky, reach the arms overhead, and press the palms firmly together to open the chest.

2. On an exhale, fold forward, reaching the hands toward the feet, clasping the big toes with the first two fingers, and pulling the shoulder blades down and back.

3. On an inhale, look up and lengthen the crown of the head toward the horizon, opening the chest. Press down with the toes while pulling up with the fingers.

4. On an exhale, pull yourself into a forward fold, with the elbows reaching out toward each side to create a straight line from the left elbow across the upper back to the right elbow. Keep the wrists lifted and in line with the elbows. Keep the thumbs tucked in or touching the fingertips instead of pushing them down into the floor.

5. Engage the inner thighs toward the midline to lift the pelvic floor and engage mula bandha. Lift the belly to engage uddiyana bandha. This will assist in pelvic tilt and support the lower-lumbar area during the compressive nature of the fold. Keep the chin locked to engage jalandhara bandha. This will aid in blood pressure control because blood moves into the head during standing forward folds.

Modifications

- To ease the hamstring stretch, bend the knees generously.
- Place the forehead or hands on blocks to help to maintain spinal extension in the forward fold.

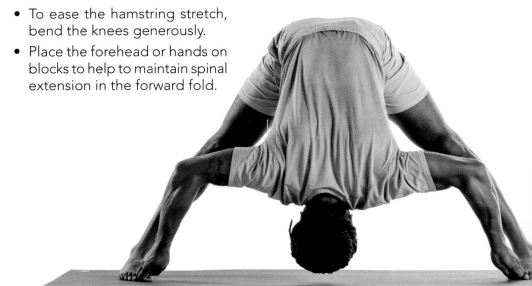

SAMAKONASANA

(sah-ma-cohn-AHS-anna)

sama = same   kona = angle   asana = pose

HORIZONTAL SPLITS

First drishti: nasikagra—tip of the nose

1. From prasarita padottanasana D (page 76), on an inhale, look up halfway to extend the spine, and then on an exhale, place both hands to the center of the mat and begin to slide the feet apart from one another, directly out to the sides. Both legs and the hips should stay in one line. If possible, sit on the ground while pressing the hands into the mat or dropping onto the elbows.

2. Keep the legs actively squeezing toward each other, with the feet pressing down to engage mula bandha. Keep the pressure of the feet on the ground to support the stability of the stretch. Uddiyana bandha will help to maintain the length in the spine and isolate the opening of the fold into the hip socket. Keep the throat locked to maintain a controlled breath.

Modification

Use a block or blocks to bring the floor closer to meet the hands.

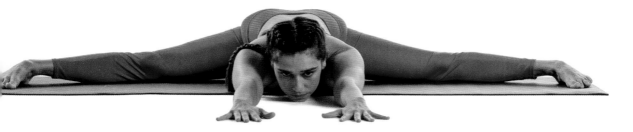

HANUMANASANA

(hah-new-mahn-AHS-anna)

hanuman = monkey king   asana = pose

CLASSIC SPLITS

First drishti: nasikagra—tip of the nose

1. From samakonasana (page 77), on an inhale, place both hands on the ground to lift the torso, and rotate the body to face the right leg. The right leg is extended straight out in front of the body, while the left leg is extended straight behind, creating one line with the legs.

2. On an exhale, slide the legs farther apart until both legs are firmly on the ground.

3. On an inhale, lengthen the spine and reach both arms overhead, touching the palms together in the center. On an exhale, fold forward over the right leg, bringing the hands toward the foot and the forehead toward the shin.

4. Hold for as long as needed, then repeat on the other side.

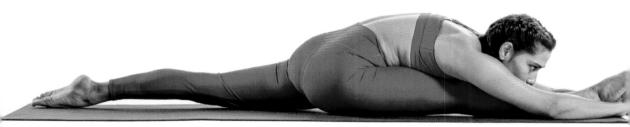

Modifications

- To ease the front leg hamstring stretch, use a block under the front thigh to support the leg and the process of relaxing without overstretching (see figure *a*).
- To focus on opening the hip of the back leg, bend the front knee generously (see figure *b*).
- Use blocks under both hands to support the body and provide grounding (see figure *c*).

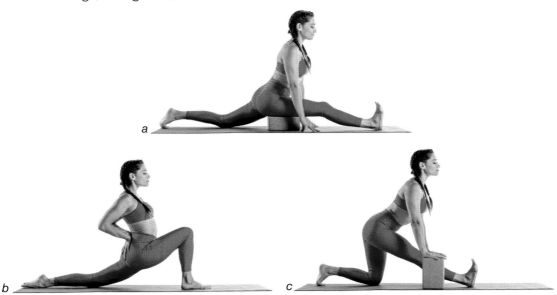

a

b

c

UPAVISTHA KONASANA VARIATION

(oo-pah-VEES-tah cohn-AHS-anna)

upavistha = seated   kona = angle   asana = pose

SEATED WIDE-ANGLE POSE

First drishti: nasikagra—tip of the nose

1. From hanumanasana (left side) (page 78), on an inhale, return to an upright seated position, and then on an exhale turn toward the side of the mat with both legs extended at equal angles from the torso.

2. On an inhale, raise both arms overhead, lengthening both sides of the body.

3. On an exhale, fold forward between the legs, leading with the heart. Maintain the extension of the spine by keeping the head up and changing the gaze to look forward. Engage the bandhas to support the weight of the torso, keeping the spine as straight as possible so that the bottom of the ribs reach the ground before the chest and head.

4. To add a side stretch on an inhale, lift the right arm toward the sky to lengthen the side body. On an exhale, reach the right hand toward the left foot, allowing the left shoulder to slide in front of the left thigh. Reach out through the right heel to ground the leg and increase the side stretch. Avoid collapsing the chest into a forward fold; instead, turn the front of the chest toward the sky to keep the stretch in the side body. Hold for as long as needed, then repeat on the other side.

Modification

If the hip flexors, inner thighs, or hamstrings are tight, do not fold forward. Instead, place the hands on the ground behind the hips and focus on sitting tall and finding the extension of the spine through the base of the sacrum.

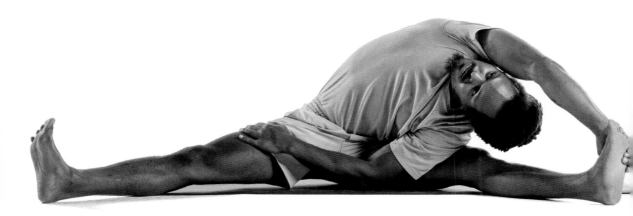

MULA BANDHA CHECKUP

(moo-lah bahn-dah)

mula = root   bandha = lock   checkup = to lift off the floor

STRADDLE PRESS

First drishti: nasikagra—tip of the nose

1. From upavistha konasana variation (page 80), on an inhale, return to an upright seated position.

2. On an exhale, place the hands on either side of the left leg, framing the knee. Take a small forward fold over the left leg, engaging the uddiyana bandha and mula bandha strongly.

3. On an inhale, press the hands into the ground to lift both legs off the ground in the straddle position. Keep the muscles of the face and jaw relaxed. Hold for as long as needed, then repeat on the other side. It is the strong engagement of the mula bandha and the lower abdominals that will lift the legs and hold them in the straddle position.

Modifications

- Use blocks under the hands to provide space to lift into.
- Lift only one or both legs, keeping the hips on the floor.
- Lift only the hips, keeping both heels on the floor.

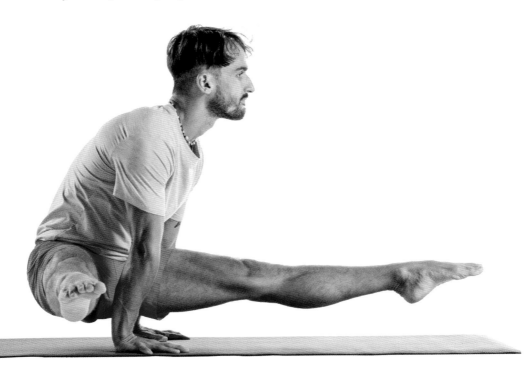

PARSVOTTANASANA

(parsh-voh-tahn-AHS-anna)

parsva = side   ut = intense   tan = stretch   asana = pose

INTENSE SIDE STRETCH POSTURE

PYRAMID POSE

Fifth drishti: padhayoragrai—toes

1. From uttanasana (page 70), bring the arms behind the body, pressing both palms together with the fingers pointing upward in a reverse prayer position. On an inhale, lift the torso until standing, and lift the chin to look up. Keep the arms in reverse prayer position.

2. On an exhale, step one foot back about three feet (1 m), keeping it in line with the front foot. Pivot on the feet to turn around to face the back of the mat.

3. On an inhale, draw the shoulder blades to the centerline, pressing the palms firmly together and taking a small backbend to open the chest and upper back.

4. On an exhale, bend from the hips over the front leg, leading with the heart center. Reach the chin toward the shin, keeping the weight in both legs even to keep the hips even and level.

5. Draw the navel into the spine to engage uddiyana bandha even before bending forward and keep the breath in the heart space. Engage the inner thighs toward the midline to lift the pelvic floor and engage mula bandha. Maintain the soft sound of the breath through the contraction of the throat to gently apply jalandhara bandha.

6. Repeat on the other side.

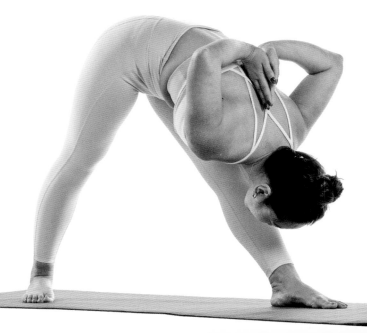

Modifications

- To aid with balance, widen the stance side to side.
- To decrease the stretch on the hamstring, place the hands on the floor, the ankle, or the shin (see figure *a*).
- To ease shoulder tension, grab opposite elbows or bring the fists together behind the back (see figure *b*).

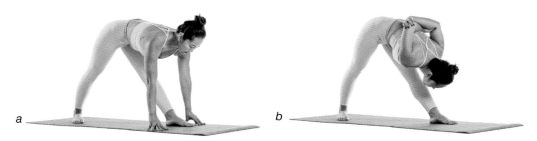

a

b

UTTHITA HASTA PADANGUSTHASANA A

(oo-TEE-tah hahs-tah pod-ang-goosh-TAHS-anna)

utthita = extended   hasta = hand
pada = foot   angustha = big toe   asana = pose

EXTENDED HAND TO BIG TOE POSTURE

Fifth drishti: padhayoragrai—toes

1. From samasthiti (page 51), on an inhale, raise the right leg, clasping the big toe with the first two fingers of the same-side hand. Keep the standing leg straight and strong, and place the other hand on the hip.
2. On an exhale, bring the head to touch the knee, taking care to roll the shoulders back and maintain the integrity of the hips.
3. Using the two-finger grip, anchor the lifted leg into the hip joint to engage uddiyana bandha and keep the breath in the heart space. Lift the pelvic floor to engage mula bandha. Maintain the soft sound of the breath through the contraction of the throat to gently apply jalandhara bandha.
4. Repeat on the other side.

Modifications

- To ease the hamstring stretch, bend the knee of the lifted leg generously.
- To aid with balance, bend the knee of the standing leg, or use a wall.

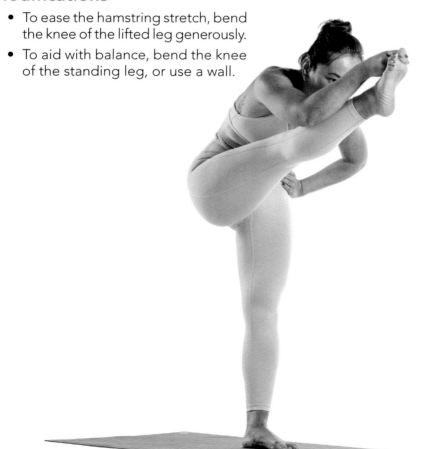

UTTHITA HASTA PADANGUSTHASANA B

(*oo-TEE-tah hahs-tah pod-ang-goosh-TAHS-anna*)

utthita = extended   hasta = hand
pada = foot   angustha = big toe   asana = pose

EXTENDED HAND TO BIG TOE POSTURE

Sixth drishti: parsva—to the right

Seventh drishti: parsva—to the left

1. From utthita hasta padangusthasana A (page 84), on an inhale, lift the head and stack the shoulders over the hips, coming into an upright position. On an exhale, open the leg to the side, maintaining the bind with the fingers. Turn the head to look in the opposite direction.

2. Keep the hips square and resist the urge to lean away from the raised leg.

3. Draw the navel into the spine to engage uddiyana bandha and keep the breath in the heart space. Lift the pelvic floor to engage mula bandha. Maintain the soft sound of the breath through the contraction of the throat to gently apply jalandhara bandha.

4. Repeat on the other side.

Modifications

- To ease the hamstring stretch, bend the knee of the lifted leg generously.
- To aid with balance, bend the knee of the standing leg, or use a wall.

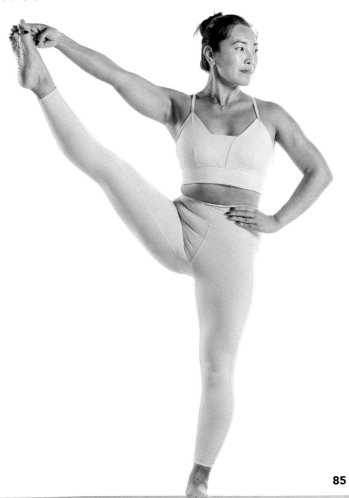

UTTHITA HASTA PADANGUSTHASANA C

(*oo-TEE-tah hahs-tah pod-ang-goosh-TAHS-anna*)

utthita = extended   hasta = hand
pada = foot   angustha = big toe   asana = pose

EXTENDED HAND TO BIG TOE POSTURE

Fifth drishti: padhayoragrai—toes

1. From utthita hasta padangusthasana B (page 85), on an inhale, bring the leg forward to the front of the mat. On an exhale, fold the head to the knee, touching once. On an inhale, lift the head up and stack the shoulders over the hips, coming into an upright position, and then release the foot from the grip. Continue to keep the leg lifted to move directly into utthita hasta padangusthasana D.

2. Draw the navel into the spine to engage uddiyana bandha and keep the breath in the heart space. Lift the pelvic floor to engage mula bandha. Maintain the soft sound of the breath through the contraction of the throat to gently apply jalandhara bandha.

3. Repeat on the other side.

Modifications

- To ease the hamstring stretch, bend the knee of the lifted leg generously.
- To aid with balance, bend the knee of the standing leg, or use a wall.

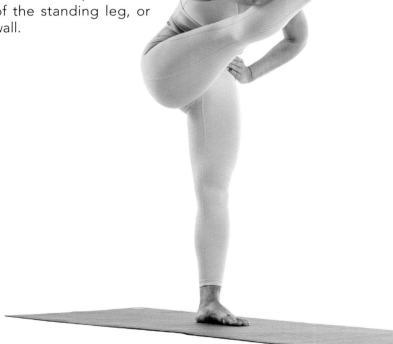

UTTHITA HASTA PADANGUSTHASANA D

(*oo-TEE-tah hahs-tah pod-ang-goosh-TAHS-anna*)

utthita = extended   hasta = hand
pada = foot   angustha = big toe   asana = pose

EXTENDED HAND TO BIG TOE POSTURE

Fifth drishti: padhayoragrai—toes

1. From utthita hasta padangusthasana C (page 86), hold the leg extended in front of the body as high as possible while keeping the shoulders stacked over the hips and the spine erect. Resist the urge to lean back in order to lift the leg. Keep both legs straight and strong.

2. Draw the navel into the spine to engage uddiyana bandha and keep the breath in the heart space. Lift the pelvic floor to engage mula bandha. Maintain the soft sound of the breath through the contraction of the throat to gently apply jalandhara bandha.

3. Repeat on the other side.

Modifications

- To ease the hamstring stretch, bend the knee of the lifted leg generously.

- To aid with balance, bend the knee of the standing leg, or use a wall.

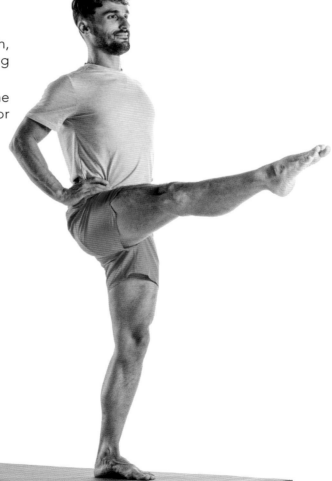

ARDHA PADMA PADMOTTANASANA

(ARD-hah PAHD-ma pahd-mo-tahn-AHS-anna)

ardha = half   padma = lotus   pada = foot   asana = pose

HALF-BOUND STANDING POSTURE

First drishti: nasikagra—tip of the nose

1. From utthita hasta padangusthasana D (page 87), on an exhale, place the foot of the lifted leg into the lotus position, pressing the outer edge of the top of the foot to the top of the opposite thigh. Reach the same-side arm behind the back and hold the foot with the hand (see figure *a*).

2. On an inhale, lengthen the spine, relax the hips, and support the balance of the body.

3. On an exhale, fold forward, placing the free hand on the ground to the outside of the foot of the standing leg, and bring the forehead to the knee (see figure *b*).

4. Draw the navel into the spine to engage uddiyana bandha, and keep the breath in the heart space. Lift the pelvic floor to engage mula bandha. Maintain the soft sound of the breath through the contraction of the throat to gently apply jalandhara bandha.

5. Repeat on the other side.

Modifications

- To aid with balance, bend the knee of the standing leg, or use a wall.
- To ease the hamstring stretch, bend the knee of the standing leg generously. A block can also be used if the ground is too far to touch.
- To ease shoulder tension, use a strap or towel to bind the hand and the lifted foot.

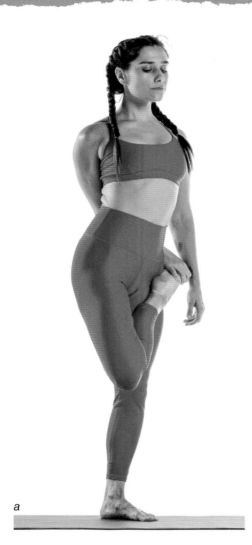

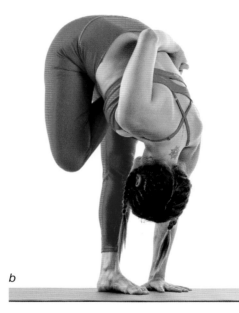

Seated Postures (Primary Series)

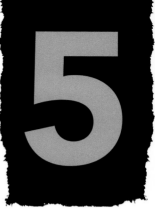

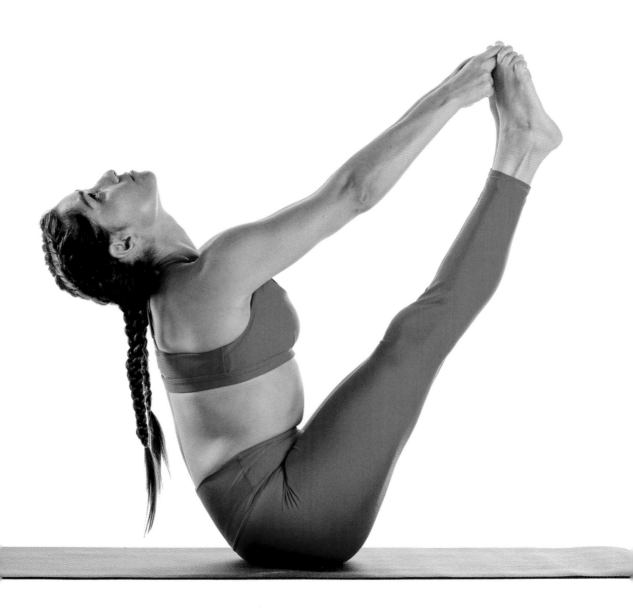

The Rocket series of poses is a modified sequence of the ashtanga vinyasa primary series, also known as *yoga chikitsa*. The classical ashtanga primary series begins after the final pose of the opening standing sequence, parsvottanasana, or pyramid pose. It starts with balancing poses, and a few more standing poses before moving on to the seated sequence, which takes up the bulk of the practice. The ashtanga primary series can be challenging for many students because of the deep forward folding and hip opening required throughout the seated sequence. Rocket yoga is a modified version of that practice that removes many of the positions that could cause injury while still maintaining the physicality and discipline of the original series. How the poses are linked in Rocket yoga brings more fluidity into the practice, which allows for more expression from each student.

In addition, many of the modifications provided for each pose are specific to the practitioner. Depending on your strengths and where you are in your practice, you will make only the modifications that allow you to receive the most benefit from the pose. For example, if you have tight hamstrings, you will make similar modifications in all of the poses that require an intense hamstring stretch.

Some of the more advanced postures of the ashtanga primary series are omitted from the Rocket yoga repertoire. Many of the postures that have been removed work more deeply with joint manipulation and hip openings and are either not accessible to the average body or difficult to perform safely on one's own. Many of the vigorous vinyasa techniques in the seated series that require a series of jumping movements to maintain heat and balance in the body have also been removed. If you progress consciously within a dedicated yoga practice, you can add the omitted postures and vinyasas back into the series under the guidance of an experienced ashtanga yoga or Rocket teacher.

DANDASANA

(dahn-DAHS-anna)

danda = staff   asana = pose

STAFF POSE

First drishti: nasikagra—tip of the nose

Fifth drishti: padhayoragrai—toes

1. From adho mukha svanasana (page 56), on an inhale, jump through the hands to a seated position, with the hips between the hands and the legs extended straight out front.

2. Flex the feet and bring the arches of the feet to touch at the center. Press the palms down into the floor, and brace the shoulder blades to the back body. Hold for as long as needed.

3. Draw the navel into the spine to engage uddiyana bandha. Engage the inner thighs toward the midline to lift the pelvic floor and engage mula bandha. Maintain the soft sound of the breath through the contraction of the throat to gently apply jalandhara bandha.

Modification

To ease the hamstring stretch, bend the knees generously.

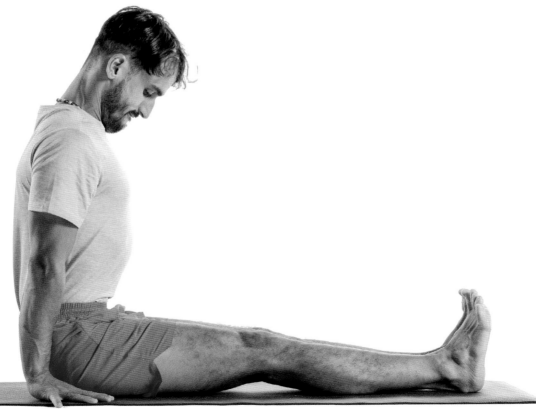

PASCHIMOTTANASANA A

(*pah-shee-moh-tahn-AHS-anna*)
paschima = back of the body
uttana = intense stretch   asana = pose

INTENSE BACK STRETCH

First drishti: nasikagra—tip of the nose

Fifth drishti: padhayoragrai—toes

1. From dandasana (page 93), on an inhale, reach the arms forward, grabbing the big toes with the first two fingers of each hand. Gently pull on the toes to extend the spine, activate the shoulders, and engage the back.

2. On an exhale, fold forward, maintaining an extended spine, and bring the chin or forehead toward the shins. Hold for as long as needed.

3. Draw the navel into the spine to engage uddiyana bandha. Engage the inner thighs toward the midline to lift the pelvic floor and engage mula bandha. Maintain the soft sound of the breath through the contraction of the throat to gently apply jalandhara bandha.

Modification

To ease the hamstring stretch, bend the knees generously.

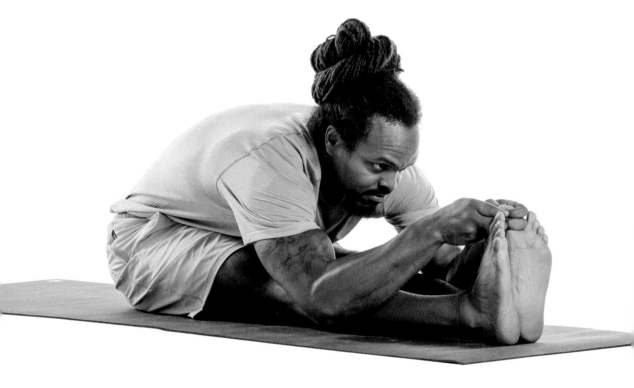

PASCHIMOTTANASANA B

(pah-shee-moh-tahn-AHS-anna)
paschima = back of the body
uttana = intense stretch   asana = pose

INTENSE BACK STRETCH

First drishti: nasikagra—tip of the nose

Fifth drishti: padhayoragrai—toes

1. From paschimottanasana A (page 94), on an inhale, extend the spine and look forward, grabbing the outer edges of the feet with the hands. Gently pull on the outer edges of the feet to extend the spine, activate the shoulders, and engage the back.

2. On an exhale, fold forward, maintaining an extended spine, and bring the chin or forehead toward the shins. Hold for as long as needed.

3. Draw the navel into the spine to engage uddiyana bandha. Engage the inner thighs toward the midline to lift the pelvic floor and engage mula bandha. Maintain the soft sound of the breath through the contraction of the throat to gently apply jalandhara bandha.

Modification

To ease the hamstring stretch, bend the knees generously.

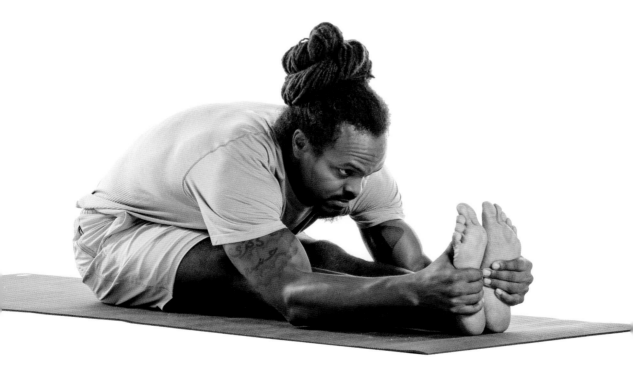

PURVOTTANASANA

(poor-voh-tahn-AHS-anna)

purva = east   uttana = intense stretch   asana = pose

INTENSE EAST STRETCH

First drishti: nasikagra—tip of the nose

1. From adho mukha svanasana (page 56), on an inhale, jump through the hands to a seated position with the hips between the hands and the legs extended straight out front.

2. On an exhale, slide the hands back behind the hips about six inches (15 cm), keeping the fingers facing forward in the same direction as the feet.

3. On an inhale, press the heels into the ground, point the toes, and lift the hips as high as possible, maintaining a straight line through the front body and keeping the legs straight.

4. Draw the navel into the spine to engage uddiyana bandha. Engage the inner thighs toward the midline to lift the pelvic floor and engage mula bandha. If possible, lift the chin for an extension through the neck.

5. Hold for as long as needed.

Modifications

- Keep the feet flat on the ground, bend the knees, and lift the hips into a reverse tabletop pose (see smaller figure).

- If there is too much tension in the neck to look up, gaze down the front body toward the knees or the feet.

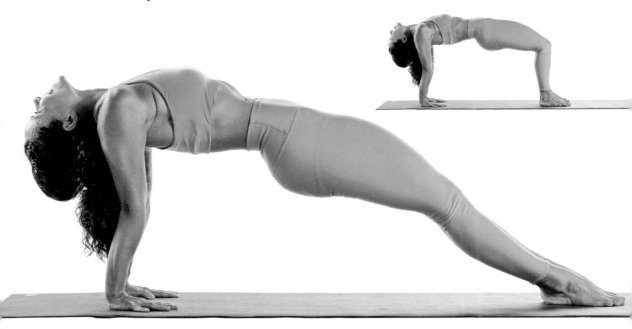

ARDHA BADDHA PADMA PASCHIMOTTANASANA

(AR-dah BAHD-ah PAHD-mah pah-shee-moh-tahn-AHS-anna)

ardha = half   baddha = bound
padma = foot   paschima = back of the body
uttana = intense stretch   asana = pose

HALF-BOUND LOTUS FORWARD FOLD

First drishti: nasikagra—tip of the nose

Fifth drishti: padhayoragrai—toes

1. From adho mukha svanasana (page 56), on an inhale, jump through the hands to a seated position with the hips between the hands and the legs extended straight out front.

2. On an exhale, bring the left foot to the lotus position, resting the outside of the foot as high as possible on the opposite thigh.

3. On an inhale, reach the left arm behind the back to grab the left foot with the left hand. Reach the right arm forward to grab the outer edge of the right foot.

4. On an exhale, fold forward.

5. Draw the navel into the spine to engage uddiyana bandha. Engage the inner thighs toward the midline to lift the pelvic floor and engage mula bandha. Maintain the soft sound of the breath through the contraction of the throat to gently apply jalandhara bandha.

6. Hold for as long as needed, then repeat on the other side.

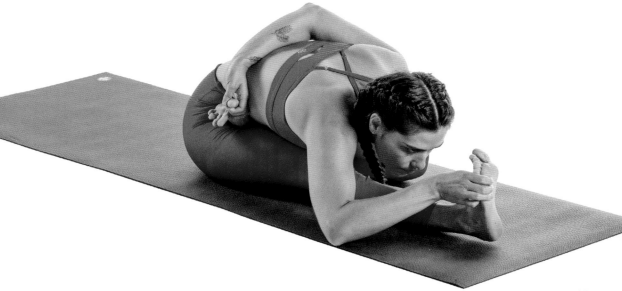

(continued)

Modifications

- To ease the hamstring stretch, bend the knees generously.
- If bringing the foot into the half lotus position is not possible, bring the sole of the right foot to the inner thigh of the left leg, resting the entire foot and leg on the ground.
- If binding around the back is not possible, use a towel or strap to close the distance between the foot and the hand (see figure).

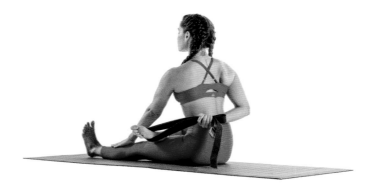

TRIANGA MUKHAIKAPADA PASCHIMOTTANASANA

(tree-AHN-gah mook-ah-pahd-ah pah-shee-moh-tahn-AHS-anna)

triang = three limbs   mukha = face   eka = one
pada = foot   paschima = back of the body
uttana = intense stretch   asana = pose

ONE-LEG FOLDED FORWARD BEND

First drishti: nasikagra—tip of the nose

Fifth drishti: padhayoragrai—toes

1. From adho mukha svanasana (page 56), on an inhale, jump through the hands to a seated position with the hips between the hands and the legs extended straight out front.
2. On an exhale, place the right foot outside of the right hip, keeping both knees together at the centerline. Try to keep both sitz bones equally on the ground.
3. On an inhale, reach both hands toward the flexed left foot, lengthening the spine.
4. On an exhale, fold forward.
5. Draw the navel into the spine to engage uddiyana bandha. Engage the inner thighs toward the midline to lift the pelvic floor and engage mula bandha. Maintain the soft sound of the breath through the contraction of the throat to gently apply jalandhara bandha.
6. Hold for as long as possible, then repeat on the other side.

Modification

To lessen internal rotation on the bent leg and ease knee pressure, place a block under the seat on the same side as the bent leg.

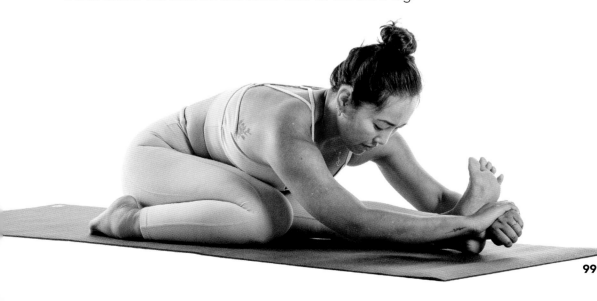

JANU SIRSASANA A AND B
(JAH-noo sheer-SHAHS-anna)
janu = knee   shirsha = head   asana = pose

HEAD TO KNEE POSE

First drishti: nasikagra—tip of the nose
Fifth drishti: padhayoragrai—toes

1. From adho mukha svanasana (page 56), on an inhale, jump through the hands to a seated position with the hips between the hands and the legs extended straight out front.
2. On an exhale, bring the sole of the right foot to the inner thigh of the left leg, resting the entire foot and leg on the ground.
3. On an inhale, reach both hands toward the flexed left foot, lengthening the spine.
4. On an exhale, fold forward. Hold for as long as needed. This is janu sirsasana A (see figure *a*).
5. To move directly into janu sirsasana B, on an inhale look up and extend the spine.
6. On an exhale, release the hands from the foot, and lift the hips to sit on top of the right heel, putting pressure on the area of the mula bandha.
7. On an inhale, reach both hands toward the flexed left foot, lengthening the spine (see figure *b*).
8. On an exhale, fold forward.
9. Draw the navel into the spine to engage uddiyana bandha. Engage the inner thighs toward the midline to lift the pelvic floor and engage mula bandha. Maintain the soft sound of the breath through the contraction of the throat to gently apply jalandhara bandha.
10. Hold for as long as needed, then repeat on the other side by doing janu sirsasana A and then B.

Modification

To ease the hamstring stretch, bend the extended leg.

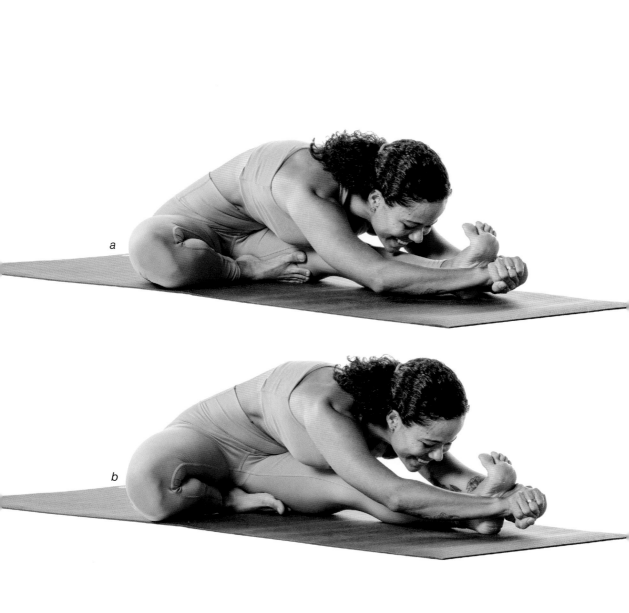

a

b

JANU SIRSASANA C
(JAH-noo sheer-SHAHS-anna)

janu = knee   shirsha = head   asana = pose

HEAD TO KNEE POSE

First drishti: nasikagra—tip of the nose

Fifth drishti: padhayoragrai—toes

1. From adho mukha svanasana (page 56), on an inhale, jump through the hands to a seated position with the hips between the hands and the legs extended straight out front.
2. On an exhale, begin by moving into janu sirsasana A by bringing the sole of the right foot to the inner thigh of the left leg, resting the entire foot and leg on the ground.
3. Keeping the right knee bent, lift the entire right leg off the ground and grip the base of the right toes with the right hand from underneath the right ankle. Externally rotate the ankle and place all five toes on the ground as close to the left thigh as possible, then gently bring the right knee down to the ground.
4. On an inhale, reach both hands toward the flexed left foot, lengthening the spine.
5. On an exhale, fold forward.
6. Draw the navel into the spine to engage uddiyana bandha. Engage the inner thighs toward the midline to lift the pelvic floor and engage mula bandha. Maintain the soft sound of the breath through the contraction of the throat to gently apply jalandhara bandha.
7. Hold for as long as needed, then repeat on the other side.

Modifications

- To ease the hamstring stretch, bend the extended leg.
- If the knee floats above the ground, place a block or blanket under the knee to support it.
- If all five toes cannot touch the ground, sit on a block placed under the seat of the extended leg to create more space for the external rotation of the ankle.

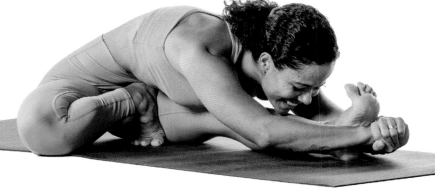

MARICHYASANA A

(mah-ree-chee-AHS-anna)

marichi = the name of a sage in Hindu mythology   asana = pose

THE POSE OF THE SAGE MARICHI

First drishti: nasikagra—tip of the nose

Fifth drishti: padhayoragrai—toes

1. From adho mukha svanasana (page 56), on an inhale, jump through the hands to a seated position with the hips between the hands and the legs extended straight out front.

2. On an exhale, bend the knee of the right leg and place the foot flat on the ground, about one hand's distance from the inner thigh of the left leg. Pull the heel of the right foot as close to the right sitz bone as possible.

3. On an inhale, reach the right arm forward, and then on an exhale, bend the elbow, reaching the arm around the right shin and below the knee. Reach the left hand behind the back and use the right hand to grab the left wrist.

4. On an inhale, lengthen the spine, and then on an exhale, fold forward, bringing the head toward the left shin.

5. Draw the navel into the spine to engage uddiyana bandha. Engage the inner thighs toward the midline to lift the pelvic floor and engage mula bandha. Maintain the soft sound of the breath through the contraction of the throat to gently apply jalandhara bandha.

6. Hold for as long as needed, then repeat on the other side.

Modification

To ease shoulder tension, use a strap or towel to bridge the gap between the hands.

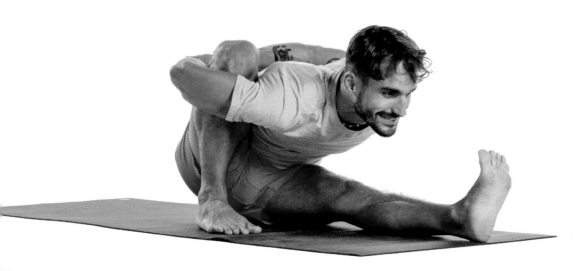

MARICHYASANA B

(mah-ree-chee-AHS-anna)

marichi = the name of a sage in Hindu mythology   asana = pose

THE POSE OF THE SAGE MARICHI

First drishti: nasikagra—tip of the nose

Fifth drishti: padhayoragrai—toes

1. From adho mukha svanasana (page 56), on an inhale, jump through the hands to a seated position with the hips between the hands and the legs extended straight out front.

2. On an exhale, bring the left foot into a half lotus position by placing the foot on top of the right thigh near the hip. Then, bend the knee of the right leg and place the foot flat on the ground, about one hand's distance from the inner thigh of the left leg. Pull the heel of the right foot as close to the right sitz bone as possible.

3. On an inhale, reach the right arm forward, and then on an exhale, bend the elbow, reaching the arm around the right shin and below the knee. Reach the left hand behind the back and use the right hand to grab the left wrist.

4. On an inhale, lengthen the spine, and then on an exhale, fold forward, bringing the head toward the ground between the knees, maintaining the extension of the spine as much as possible.

5. Draw the navel into the spine to engage uddiyana bandha. Engage the inner thighs toward the midline to lift the pelvic floor and engage mula bandha. Maintain the soft sound of the breath through the contraction of the throat to gently apply jalandhara bandha.

6. Hold for as long as needed, then repeat on the other side.

Modification

To ease shoulder tension, use a strap or towel to bridge the gap between the hands.

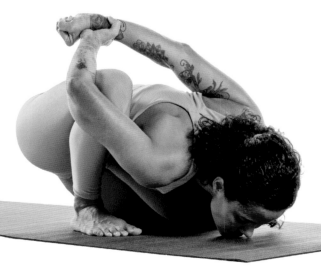

MARICHYASANA C

(mah-ree-chee-AHS-anna)

marichi = the name of a sage in Hindu mythology   asana = pose

THE POSE OF THE SAGE MARICHI

First drishti: nasikagra—tip of the nose

Fifth drishti: padhayoragrai—toes

1. From adho mukha svanasana (page 56), on an inhale, jump through the hands to a seated position with the hips between the hands and the legs extended straight out front.

2. On an exhale, bend the knee of the right leg and place the foot flat on the ground about one hand's distance from the inner thigh of the left leg. Pull the heel of the right foot as close to the right sitz bone as possible.

3. On an inhale, reach the right arm up, then on an exhale, twist toward the right side, placing the right hand on the ground behind the hips. Bring the right knee to the outside of the left armpit, wrapping the left arm around the bent right leg to reach toward the back. Reach the right hand behind the back toward the left hand, and then use the left hand to grab the right wrist.

4. Draw the navel into the spine to engage uddiyana bandha. Engage the inner thighs toward the midline to lift the pelvic floor and engage mula bandha. Maintain the soft sound of the breath through the contraction of the throat to gently apply jalandhara bandha.

5. Hold for as long as needed, then repeat on the other side.

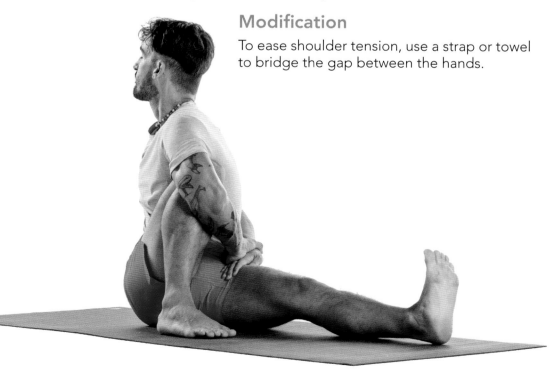

Modification

To ease shoulder tension, use a strap or towel to bridge the gap between the hands.

MARICHYASANA D

(*mah-ree-chee-AHS-anna*)

marichi = the name of a sage in Hindu mythology   asana = pose

THE POSE OF THE SAGE MARICHI

First drishti: nasikagra—tip of the nose

Fifth drishti: padhayoragrai—toes

1. From adho mukha svanasana (page 56), on an inhale, jump through the hands to a seated position with the hips between the hands and the legs extended straight out front.

2. On an exhale, bring the left foot into a half lotus position by placing the foot on top of the right thigh near the hip. Then, bend the knee of the right leg and place the foot flat on the ground, about one hand's distance from the inner thigh of the left leg. Pull the heel of the right foot as close to the right sitz bone as possible.

3. On an inhale, reach the right arm up, then on an exhale, twist toward the right side, placing the right hand on the ground behind the hips. Bring the right knee to the outside of the left armpit, wrapping the left arm around the bent right leg to reach toward the back. Reach the right hand behind the back toward the left hand, and then use the left hand to grab the right wrist.

4. Draw the navel into the spine to engage uddiyana bandha. Engage the inner thighs toward the midline to lift the pelvic floor and engage mula bandha. Maintain the soft sound of the breath through the contraction of the throat to gently apply jalandhara bandha.

5. Hold for as long as needed, then repeat on the other side.

Modification

To ease shoulder tension, use a strap or towel to bridge the gap between the hands.

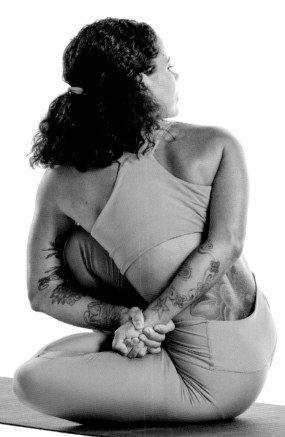

NAVASANA/LOLASANA

(*nah-VAHS-anna*) (*loh-LAHS-anna*)

nava = boat   asana = pose

BOAT POSE

First drishti: nasikagra—tip of the nose

Fifth drishti: padhayoragrai—toes

1. From adho mukha svanasana (page 56), on an inhale, jump through the hands to a seated position with the hips between the hands and the legs lifted straight and the feet at the same level as the eyes. Reach the hands forward toward the feet, palms facing inward toward one another. This is navasana (see figure a).

2. Hold for five breaths, and then bring both hands to the ground beside the hips. Cross the legs at the ankles, and keep the feet off the floor.

3. On an inhale, press the hands into the ground, and lift the hips (see figure b). On an exhale, return the hips to the ground, and bring the legs back into the initial position. This is lolasana.

4. Draw the navel into the spine to engage uddiyana bandha. Engage the inner thighs toward the midline to lift the pelvic floor and engage mula bandha. Maintain the soft sound of the breath through the contraction of the throat to gently apply jalandhara bandha.

5. Repeat this movement three to five times.

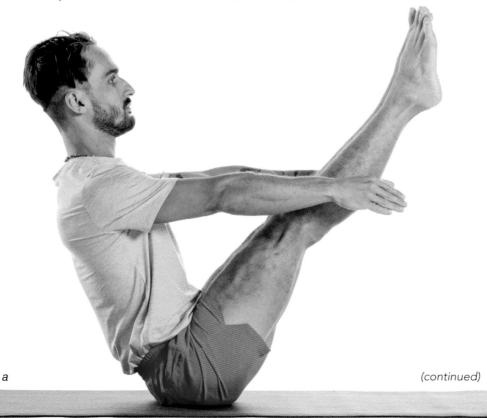

a

(continued)

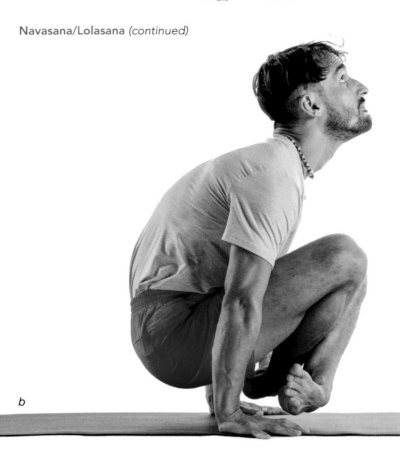

b

Modifications

- To ease the hamstring stretch, bend both knees, keeping the shins parallel to the ground (see figure *a*).
- To decrease abdominal work, bend the knees and use the hands to hold behind the thighs (see figure *b*).
- Use a block under each hand for the lift (see figure *c*).

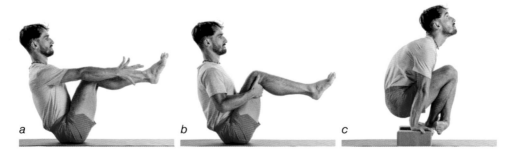

a   b   c

BHUJAPIDASANA

(BOO-jah-pee-DAHS-ahna)

bhuja = shoulder   pida = pressure   asana = pose

SHOULDER PRESSURE POSE

First drishti: nasikagra—tip of the nose

1. From adho mukha svanasana (page 56), jump the feet forward and outside of the hands. Continue to walk the feet forward, or move the hands behind the heels of the feet. Begin to sit the hips low into the pose, with the back of the thighs resting on the shelf of the triceps of the arms.

2. Balancing on the hands, lift both feet off the ground, crossing the left ankle over the right, and keeping both feet flexed. Advanced students can jump directly from adho mukha svanasana into this stage of the pose.

3. On an exhale, bring the chin to the mat while keeping both feet off the floor. If you cannot reach your chin to the floor, bring the top of the head to the floor to begin and slowly work toward bringing the chin down.

4. Draw the navel into the spine to engage uddiyana bandha. Engage the inner thighs toward the midline to lift the pelvic floor and engage mula bandha. Maintain the soft sound of the breath through the contraction of the throat to gently apply jalandhara bandha.

5. Stay here for five breaths.

6. On an inhale, come out of the pose in the same way you moved into it, maintaining the same integrity of movement. Move the legs through bakasana, then jump back directly into chaturanga dandasana. Try not to bring the feet down to the ground at any time.

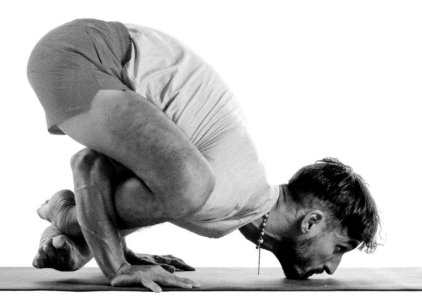

KURMASANA

(*koor-MAHS-ahna*)

kurma = tortoise   asana = pose

TORTOISE POSE

First drishti: nasikagra—tip of the nose

1. From adho mukha svanasana (page 56), jump the feet forward and outside of the hands. Continue to walk the feet forward, or move the hands behind the heels of the feet. Begin to sit the hips low into the pose, with the back of the thighs resting on the shelf of the triceps of the arms.

2. Bring the hips all the way down onto the ground. Extend the arms directly out to the side or slightly reaching back in a V-shape. Extend the legs straight forward on top of the arms, pointing the toes and lifting the feet off the ground by straightening the legs strongly.

3. Draw the navel into the spine to engage uddiyana bandha. Engage the inner thighs toward the midline to lift the pelvic floor and engage mula bandha. Maintain the soft sound of the breath through the contraction of the throat to gently apply jalandhara bandha.

4. Stay here for five breaths, then move directly into supta kurmasana.

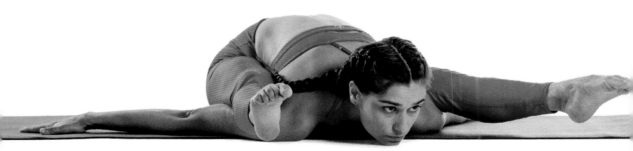

SUPTA KURMASANA

(SOOP-tah koor-MAHS-ahna)

supta = reclined   kurma = tortoise   asana = pose

SLEEPING TORTOISE POSE

First drishti: nasikagra—tip of the nose

1. From kurmasana (page 110), internally rotate the arms and bring the hands together across the lower back.

2. Bring the feet to cross behind the head, starting with the left leg first, then bringing the right leg behind the left. Point the toes. Press the head back into the feet and broaden across the collarbones.

3. Draw the navel into the spine to engage uddiyana bandha and then lift the pelvic floor to engage mula bandha.

4. Stay here for five breaths.

5. Keeping the legs crossed behind the head, unclasp the hands and bring both hands down the mat, shoulder-width apart. Press into the hands to lift up.

6. On an inhale, uncross the ankles and straighten the legs into titibhasana, then on an exhale, move the legs through bakasana and jump back into chaturanga dandasana.

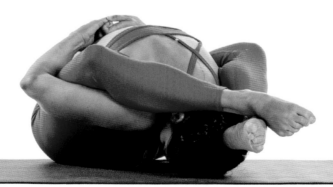

GARBA PIDASANA

(gar-bah pee-DAHS-ahna)

garba = womb   pinda = embryo   asana = pose

EMBRYO IN WOMB POSE

First drishti: nasikagra—tip of the nose

1. From adho mukha svanasana (page 56), on an inhale, jump through the hands to a seated position with the hips between the hands and the legs extended straight out front.
2. Bring your legs into a full lotus position, drawing the right foot in first, then crossing the left shin over the right.
3. In the space between your upper calf and your thighs, push your arms through up to the elbow joint. You may find it easier to start with your right arm, but it's not important here which arm you start with. If you have trouble, you can roll up your leggings or apply some oil or water to your arms to facilitate this movement.
4. Once your arms are through, bend them deeply at the elbow and reach your hands toward your ears or the sides of your face. You will need to stay balanced here.
5. Hold for five breaths.
6. Bring both hands toward the crown of the head, then begin to roll back and forth, up and down the length of the spine. You want to roll back and forth nine times in a circle, eventually ending up back at the front of your mat. Once at the front of your mat, go directly into kukkutasana.

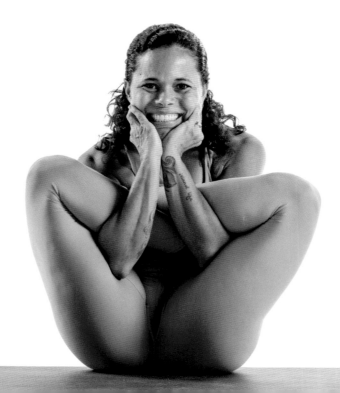

KUKKUTASANA

(koo-koo-TAHS-ahna)

kukku = rooster   asana = pose

ROOSTER POSE

First drishti: nasikagra—tip of the nose

1. From garba pidasana (page 112), press your hands down into the mat, shoulder-width apart.
2. Lean forward, and lift the rest of your body off the floor. Keep drawing the legs up toward your chest.
3. Hold for five breaths.

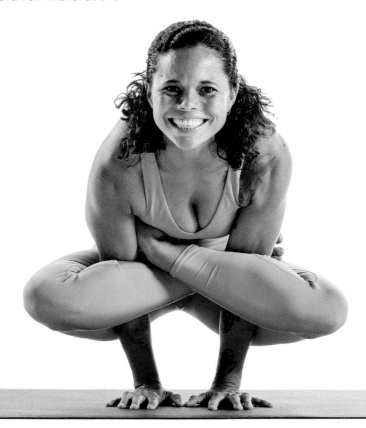

BADDHA KONASANA A AND B
(BAHD-ah cohn-AHS-anna)
badha = bound   kona = angle   asana = pose

BOUND ANGLE POSE

COBBLER'S POSE

BUTTERFLY POSE

First drishti: nasikagra—tip of the nose

1. From adho mukha svanasana (page 56), on an inhale, jump through the hands to a seated position with the hips between the hands and the legs extended straight out front.
2. On an exhale, bend both knees, bringing the soles of the feet together in the center and pulling the heels as close as possible toward the pubic bone. Use the hands to hold the feet or ankles.
3. On an inhale, extend the spine, then on an exhale, fold forward, bringing the chin toward the floor in front of the feet.
4. Draw the navel into the spine to engage uddiyana bandha. Engage the inner thighs toward the midline to lift the pelvic floor and engage mula bandha. Maintain the soft sound of the breath through the contraction of the throat to gently apply jalandhara bandha. This is baddha konasana A (see figure *a*).
5. Hold for as long as needed.
6. On an inhale, return to an upright seat. Draw the belly into the spine and bring the spine into flexion by curling into yourself. Bring the forehead to touch the arches of the feet.
7. Draw the navel into the spine to engage uddiyana bandha. Engage the inner thighs toward the midline to lift the pelvic floor and engage mula bandha. Maintain the soft sound of the breath through the contraction of the throat to gently apply jalandhara bandha. This is baddha konasana B (see figure *b*).
8. Hold for as long as needed.

Modification

To ease hip opening, place blocks under each knee, or simply sit up straight instead of folding forward.

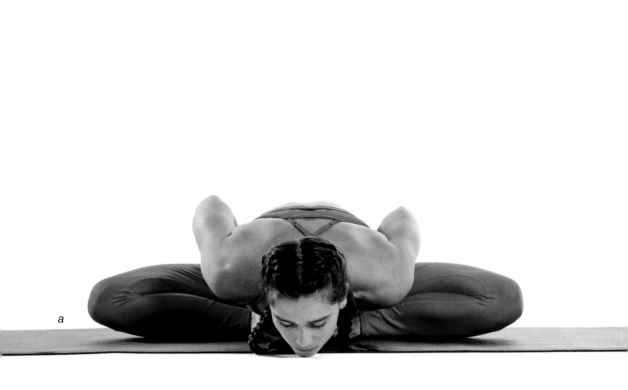

a

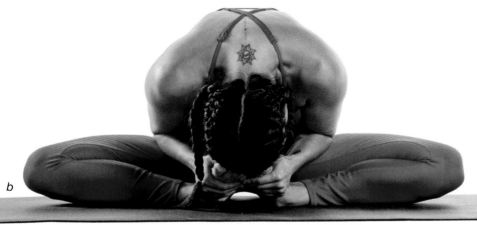

b

UPAVISTHA KONASANA A AND B

(OO-pah-vish-tah cohn-AHS-anna)

upavistha = open   kona = angle   asana = pose

WIDE-ANGLE SEATED FORWARD BEND

First drishti: nasikagra—tip of the nose

1. From adho mukha svanasana (page 56), on an inhale, jump through the hands to a seated position with the hips between the hands and the legs extended straight out front.
2. On an exhale, open the legs wide to about 90 degrees, keeping the legs straight.
3. On an inhale, grab the big toes with the first two fingers of each hand and extend the spine (see figure *a*).
4. On an exhale, fold forward, bringing the chest and chin to the ground. This is upavishtha konasana A.
5. Hold for five breaths.
6. On an inhale, look up and lengthen the spine. On an exhale, release the toes and sit tall.
7. On an inhale, lift the legs, keeping them straight and catching the outer edge of the feet with the hands. Stay balanced on the sitz bones, and lift the chin to gaze upward. This is upavishtha konasana B (see figure *b*).
8. Hold for five breaths.
9. Draw the navel into the spine to engage uddiyana bandha. Engage the inner thighs toward the midline to lift the pelvic floor and engage mula bandha. Maintain the soft sound of the breath through the contraction of the throat to gently apply jalandhara bandha.

Modification

To ease the hamstring stretch, bend the knees generously.

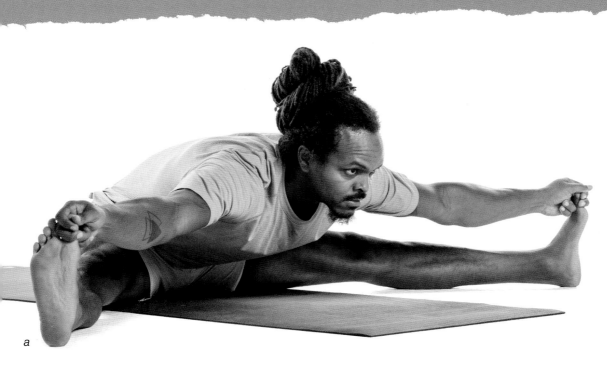

a

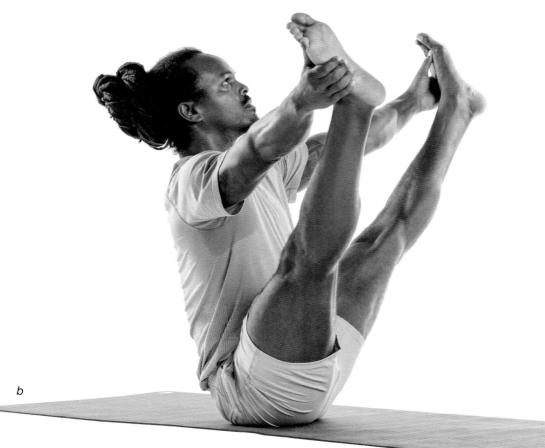

b

117

SUPTA KONASANA A AND B
(SOOP-tah cohn-AHS-anna)
supta = reclining   kona = angle   asana = pose

RECLINING ANGLE POSE

First drishti: nasikagra—tip of the nose

Fifth drishti: padhayoragrai—toes

1. From adho mukha svanasana (page 56), on an inhale, jump through the hands to a seated position with the hips between the hands and the legs extended straight out front.
2. On an exhale, lie flat on your back.
3. On an inhale, raise both legs overhead, spreading the legs wide and setting the feet on the floor behind the head. Keep both legs straight, and on an exhale, grab the big toes with the first two fingers of each hand. This is supta konasana A (see figure a).
4. Hold for five breaths.
5. On an inhale, keep holding the big toes and rock up to balance on the sitz bones (see figure b).
6. On an exhale, flex both feet hard and allow the body to fall forward, landing on the calves and bringing the chin near the ground. This is supta konasana B (see figure c).
7. Draw the navel into the spine to engage uddiyana bandha. Engage the inner thighs toward the midline to lift the pelvic floor and engage mula bandha. Maintain the soft sound of the breath through the contraction of the throat to gently apply jalandhara bandha.

Modification

To ease the hamstring stretch, bend the knees generously.

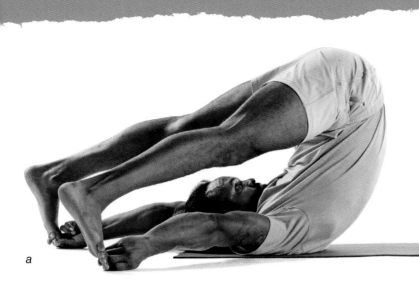

a

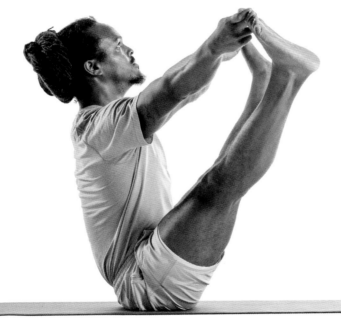

b

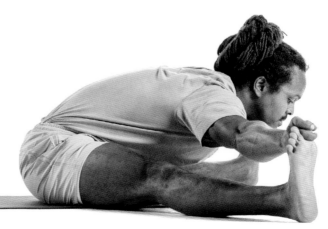

c

SUPTA PADANGUSTHASANA

(SOOP-tah pod-ang-goosh-TAHS-anna)
supta = reclining   pada = foot
angustha = big toe   asana = pose

RECLINING BIG TOE POSTURE

First drishti: nasikagra—tip of the nose

Fifth drishti: padhayoragrai—toes

1. From adho mukha svanasana (page 56), on an inhale, jump through the hands to a seated position with the hips between the hands and the legs extended straight out front.
2. On an exhale, lie flat on your back.
3. On an inhale, lift the right leg, and use the first two fingers of the right hand to catch the right big toe, keeping the leg straight. Keep the left arm straight, pressing the left hand down onto the top of the left thigh.
4. On an exhale, lift the head and bring the forehead near the right knee (see figure a). Hold for five breaths.
5. On an inhale, rest the head on the ground. On an exhale, open the right leg to the right side, and turn the head to look over the left shoulder (see figure b).
6. Hold for five breaths.
7. On an inhale, bring the leg back to center. On an exhale, touch the head to the left knee once.
8. On an inhale, rest the head on the ground, and repeat on the other side.
9. Draw the navel into the spine to engage uddiyana bandha. Engage the inner thighs toward the midline to lift the pelvic floor and engage mula bandha. Maintain the soft sound of the breath through the contraction of the throat to gently apply jalandhara bandha.

Modification

To ease the hamstring stretch, bend the knees generously, or use a strap or towel to reach the foot.

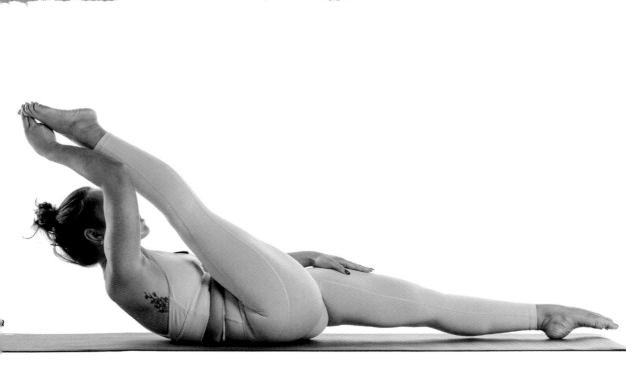

a

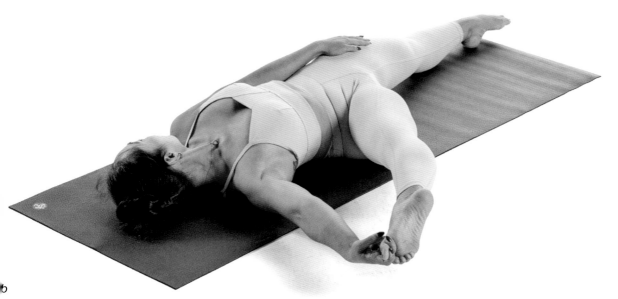

b

121

UBHAYA PADANGUSTHASANA

(oo-BAI-yah pod-ang-goosh-TAHS-anna)

ubhaya = both   pada = foot   angustha = big toe   asana = pose

BOTH BIG TOES POSE

First drishti: nasikagra—tip of the nose

Fifth drishti: padhayoragrai—toes

1. From adho mukha svanasana (page 56), on an inhale, jump through the hands to a seated position with the hips between the hands and the legs extended straight out front.

2. On an exhale, lie flat on your back.

3. On an inhale, raise both legs overhead, keeping the legs together and setting the feet on the floor behind the head. Keep both legs straight, and on an exhale, grab the big toes with the first two fingers of each hand (see figure *a*).

4. On an inhale, keep holding the big toes, and rock up to balance on the sitz bones (see figure *b*).

5. Hold for five breaths.

6. Draw the navel into the spine to engage uddiyana bandha. Engage the inner thighs toward the midline to lift the pelvic floor and engage mula bandha. Maintain the soft sound of the breath through the contraction of the throat to gently apply jalandhara bandha.

Modification

To ease the hamstring stretch, bend the knees generously.

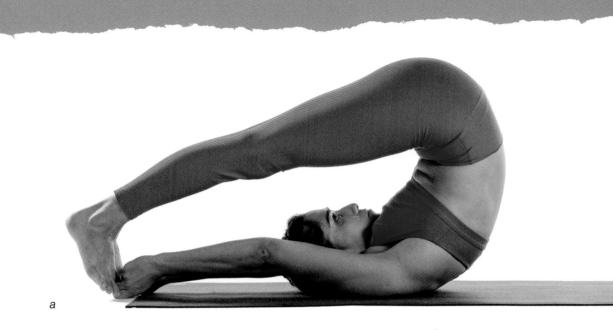

a

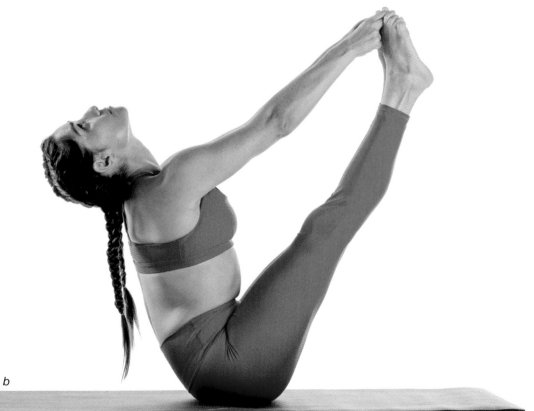

b

URDHVA MUKHA PASCHIMOTTANASANA

(OORD-vah MOO-kah pah-shee-moh-tahn-AHS-anna)

urdhva = upward   mukha = face   paschima = back of the body

uttana = intense stretch   asana = pose

UPWARD-FACING FORWARD STRETCH POSE

First drishti: nasikagra—tip of the nose

1. From adho mukha svanasana (page 56), on an inhale, jump through the hands to a seated position with the hips between the hands and the legs extended straight out front.

2. On an exhale, lie flat on your back.

3. On an inhale, raise both legs overhead, keeping the legs together and setting the feet on the floor behind the head. Keep both legs straight, and on an exhale, grab the heels of the feet with the hands (see figure a).

4. On an inhale, catch the outer edge of the feet with the hands, and rock up to balance on the sitz bones (see figure b).

5. On an exhale, bend the elbows and bring the forehead to the shins.

6. Hold for five breaths.

7. Draw the navel into the spine to engage uddiyana bandha. Engage the inner thighs toward the midline to lift the pelvic floor and engage mula bandha. Maintain the soft sound of the breath through the contraction of the throat to gently apply jalandhara bandha.

Modification

To ease the hamstring stretch, bend the knees generously.

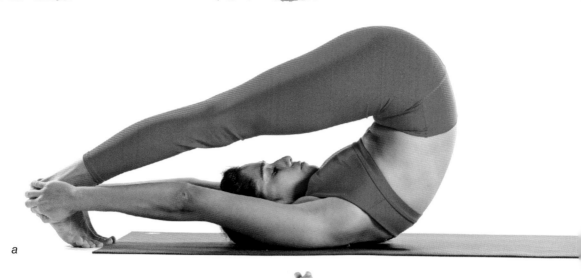

a

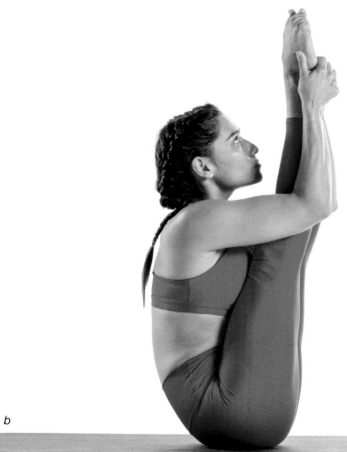

b

SETU BANDHASANA
(SAY-too BAHN-duh-AHS-uh-nuh)

setu = bridge   bandha = caught   asana = pose

BRIDGE POSE

Second drishti: bhrumadhya—between the eyebrows (third eye)

1. From adho mukha svanasana (page 56), on an inhale, jump through the hands to a seated position with the hips between the hands and the legs extended straight out front. Lie flat on your back.
2. Bend the knees and place the outer edges of the feet on the ground with the heels touching and the toes apart.
3. Put weight into your forearms to arch the back off the ground, placing the crown of the head on the ground but keeping your hips down.
4. Cross the arms across your chest and bring each hand to the opposite shoulder.
5. On an inhale, press into the outer edge of the feet and the crown of the head to lift the hips up and send the weight of the body into the legs.
6. Hold for five breaths.
7. Draw the navel into the spine to engage uddiyana bandha. Engage the inner thighs toward the midline to lift the pelvic floor and engage mula bandha.

Modification

If this pose puts an uncomfortable amount of pressure in the neck, use your hands for support as you lift or simply keep the hips on the ground.

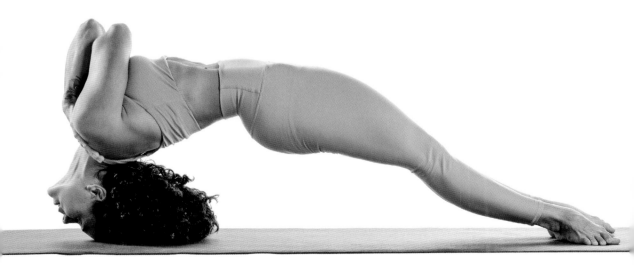

ARDHA URDHVA DHANURASANA

(ARD-ah OORD-vah dahn-you-RAHS-anna)

ardha = half   urdhva = upward   danura = wheel   asana = pose

HALF-WHEEL POSE

First drishti: nasikagra—tip of the nose

1. From adho mukha svanasana (page 56), on an inhale, jump through the hands to a seated position with the hips between the hands and the legs extended straight out front.

2. On an exhale, lie flat on your back. Bend the knees toward the sky, bringing the feet flat on the ground about hip-width apart. Bring the heels in toward the sitz bones as close as possible.

3. On an inhale, press the feet into the ground, and lift the hips as high as possible.

4. Hold for five breaths.

5. Draw the navel into the spine to engage uddiyana bandha. Engage the inner thighs toward the midline to lift the pelvic floor and engage mula bandha. Maintain the soft sound of the breath through the contraction of the throat to gently apply jalandhara bandha.

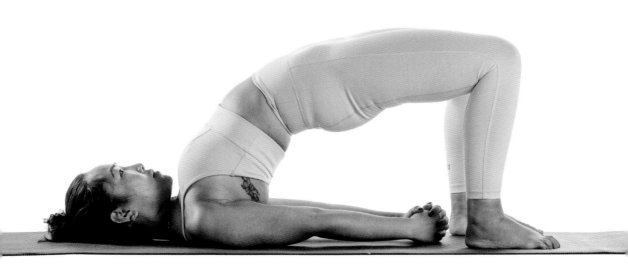

URDHVA DHANURASANA

(OORD-vah dahn-you-RAHS-anna)

urdhva = upward   danura = wheel   asana = pose

WHEEL POSE

UPWARD-FACING BOW POSE

First drishti: nasikagra–tip of the nose

1. From ardha urdhva dhanurasana (page 127), on an exhale, place the hands next to the ears with the palms on the floor and the fingers facing the shoulders.
2. On an inhale, press the feet and hands into the ground to lift the entire body into a full wheel. Lift the chin to look toward the hands.
3. Hold for five breaths.

Modification

If this pose is too difficult, use a half wheel.

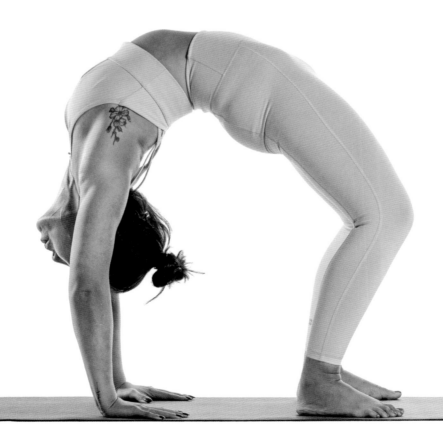

Seated Postures (Rocket Intermediate)

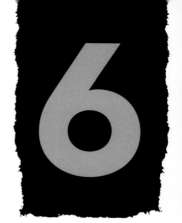

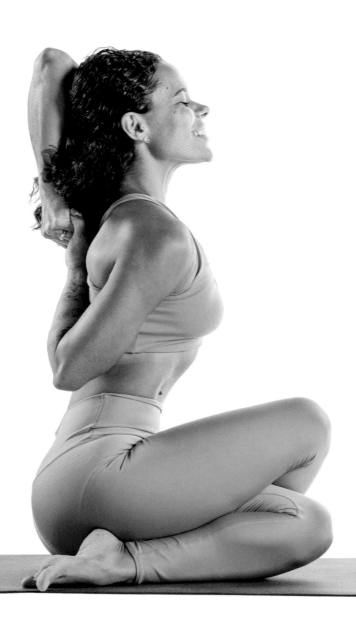

The intermediate series carries with it a different energy than the primary series. Along with more backbends come even deeper twists and hip openers as well as inversions. All together, they cleanse the nervous system of previously held patterns and bring fluidity to the physical body as well as the mind.

The poses incorporate some of the arm balances from the classical ashtanga third series to add an arm-strengthening component as well as integrating core stability before the deeper backbending sequence. The poses of the intermediate series are intentionally challenging. Many poses take the body to extreme end ranges of mobility. For this reason, few modifications are offered in this section. Knowing when your body is ready to take on these poses is up to you and the experience of a qualified teacher. Connecting with your body and being aware of the patterns in your mind as you face these challenges is the practice of yoga.

PASASANA

(pash-AHS-anna)

pasa = noose   asana = pose

NOOSE POSTURE

First drishti: nasikagra—tip of the nose

1. From adho mukha svanasana (page 56), on an inhale, jump to squat between your hands at the top of the mat; reach the heels toward the ground if possible. Keep the knees and feet firmly pressing together.

2. On an exhale, twist to the right, hooking the left elbow outside of the right thigh. Place as much of the shoulder behind the thigh that the upper arm rests on, and not just the elbow. Bring the palms into a prayer position, and lift the chest so the thumbs touch the sternum. Stay here or bind both hands behind your back, encircling both knees if possible. Allow the tailbone to drop, and lift the twist through the upper back.

3. Draw the navel into the spine to engage uddiyana bandha and deepen the twist. Engage the inner thighs toward the midline to lift the pelvic floor and engage mula bandha. Maintain the soft sound of the breath through the contraction of the throat to gently apply jalandhara bandha.

4. Hold for as long as needed, then repeat on the other side.

Modifications

- If the heels do not reach the ground, lift the heels or use a block or a rolled-up towel to support the heels.
- To lessen work in the hips and decrease the twist, squat with the legs apart and work the twisting action by hooking the elbow to the inside of the thigh.
- To help with balance, practice squatting low with a wall behind you for support.

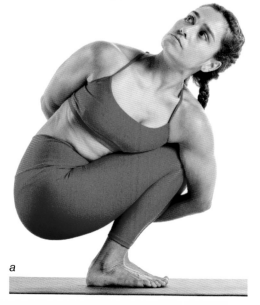

a

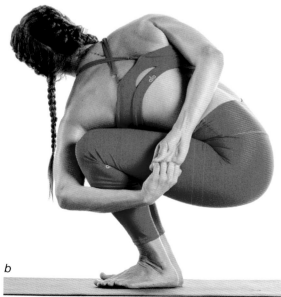

b

PARSVA BAKASANA

(PARS-vah bahk-AHS-anna)

parsva = side   baka = crane   asana = pose

SIDE CROW (CRANE) POSE

First drishti: nasikagra—tip of the nose

1. From pasasana (page 131), on an exhale, release the hands and place them shoulder-width apart at the top of the mat. Twist the lower body toward the left side so the right knee can rest atop the left elbow.

2. On an inhale, squeeze the thighs together, and shift the weight over the elbows, lifting both feet off the mat and balancing on the hands. Keep the toes and heels even as you squeeze the heels to your sitz bones. Keep the elbows stacked on top of the wrists and the hips higher than the shoulders.

3. Draw the navel into the spine to engage uddiyana bandha and stabilize the core. Engage the inner thighs toward the midline to lift the pelvic floor and engage mula bandha. This will provide a sensation of lightness in the pose. Maintain the soft sound of the breath through the contraction of the throat to gently apply jalandhara bandha.

4. Hold for as long as needed, then repeat on the other side.

Modification

To aid with balance, bring the hip of the knee that is resting atop the elbow to the other elbow, supporting the weight of the upper body across both elbows (see smaller figure).

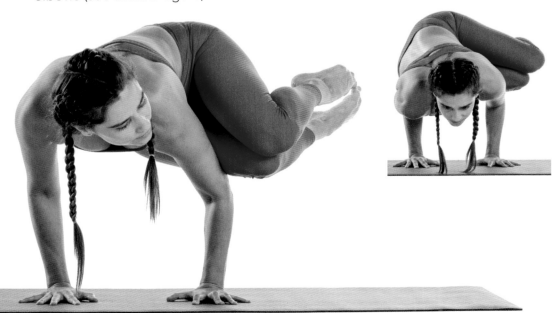

PARSVA KOUNDINYASANA

(PARS-vah cawn-din-YAHS-anna)

parsva = side   Kaundinya = an ancient Indian sage   asana = pose

SAGE KAUNDINYA'S POSE

TWISTING KARDINYA'S ONE-FOOTED POSE

First drishti: nasikagra—tip of the nose

1. From parsva bakasana (page 132), on an inhale, straighten both legs as you scissor them apart, extending the top leg toward the back of the mat and the bottom leg out to the side.

2. Draw the navel into the spine to engage uddiyana bandha and stabilize the core. Engage the inner thighs toward the midline to lift the pelvic floor and engage mula bandha. This will provide a sensation of lightness in the pose. Maintain the soft sound of the breath through the contraction of the throat to gently apply jalandhara bandha.

3. Hold for as long as needed, then repeat on the other side.

Modification

If this is too difficult, use side crow pose (page 132).

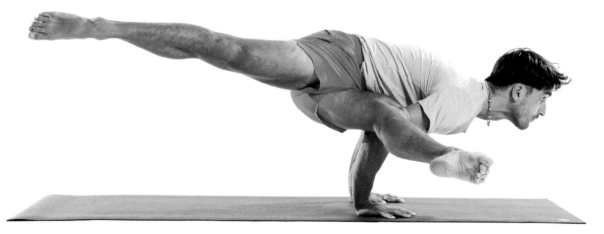

DWI PADA KOUNDINYASANA

(dvee pah-dah cawn-din-YAHS-anna)

dvee = two   pada = foot

Kaundinya = an ancient Indian sage   asana = pose

KAUNDINYA'S TWO-LEGGED POSE

First drishti: nasikagra—tip of the nose

1. From parsva koundinyasana (page 133), on an exhale, briefly return to parsva bakasana (page 132).
2. On an inhale, straighten both legs out to the side, keeping the toes touching and the hips lifted.
3. Draw the navel into the spine to engage uddiyana bandha and stabilize the core. Engage the inner thighs toward the midline to lift the pelvic floor and engage mula bandha. This will provide a sensation of lightness in the pose. Maintain the soft sound of the breath through the contraction of the throat to gently apply jalandhara bandha.
4. Hold for as long as needed, then repeat on the other side.

Modification

If this is too difficult, use side crow pose (page 132).

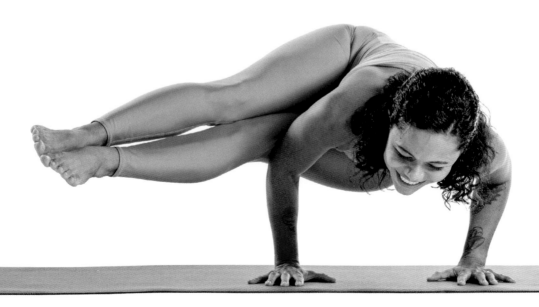

KROUNCHASANA

(krawn-CHAHS-anna)

kraunch = heron   asana = pose

HERON POSE

First drishti: nasikagra—tip of the nose

1. From adho mukha svanasana (page 56), on an inhale, jump through the hands to a seated position with the hips between the hands. The left leg is extended straight out front, the right leg is bent with the right foot outside of the hip, and the toes point to the back.

2. Keep the left leg raised throughout this movement, and clasp the left leg with both hands and pull it toward the body until it is perpendicular to the ground (see figures a and b). Keep the toes pointed.

3. Draw the navel into the spine to engage uddiyana bandha. Engage the inner thighs toward the midline to lift the pelvic floor and engage mula bandha. Maintain the soft sound of the breath through the contraction of the throat to gently apply jalandhara bandha.

4. Hold for as long as needed, then repeat on the other side.

Modification

If this is too difficult, use the one-leg folded forward bend (page 99).

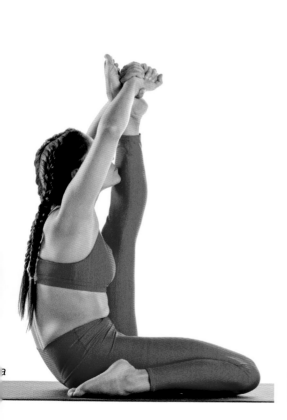

a

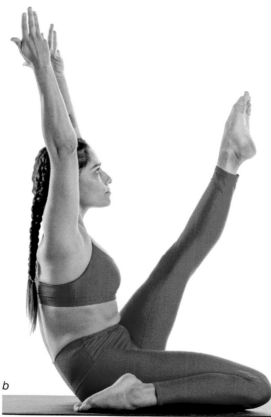

b

EKA PADA BAKASANA

(e-kah pah-dah bahk-AHS-anna)

eka = one   pada = foot   baka = crane   asana = pose

ONE-LEG CROW POSE

First drishti: nasikagra—tip of the nose

1. From krounchasana variation (page 135), on an exhale, bend the right knee, placing the right foot on the floor and hooking the right knee under the right armpit. Place the hands shoulder-width apart on the mat.

2. On an inhale, lean forward until the elbows are over the wrists, shifting the weight and balancing on the hands. The right foot leaves the ground, and the left leg lifts and extends straight back and up.

3. Draw the navel into the spine to engage uddiyana bandha and stabilize the core. Engage the inner thighs toward the midline to lift the pelvic floor and engage mula bandha. This will provide a sensation of lightness in the pose. Maintain the soft sound of the breath through the contraction of the throat to gently apply jalandhara bandha.

4. Hold for as long as needed, then repeat on the other side.

Modification

If this is too difficult, use side crow pose (page 132).

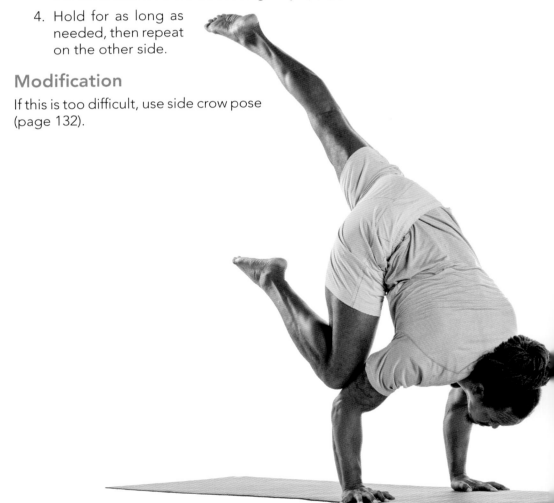

ASTAVAKRASANA

(ahsh-ta-va-KRAHS-anna)

asta = eight   vakra = bent, curved   asana = pose

EIGHT ANGLE POSE

First drishti: nasikagra—tip of the nose

1. From adho mukha svanasana (page 56), on an inhale, jump the left leg through the arms, and let the right leg wrap over the right elbow, crossing the legs at the ankles.

2. On an exhale, bend the elbows to 90 degrees, lowering the torso toward the mat, squeezing the thighs together, and extending both legs toward the right. Keep the legs parallel to the ground.

3. Draw the navel into the spine to engage uddiyana bandha and stabilize the core. Engage the inner thighs toward the midline to lift the pelvic floor and engage mula bandha. This will provide a sensation of lightness in the pose. Maintain the soft sound of the breath through the contraction of the throat to gently apply jalandhara bandha.

4. Hold for as long as needed, then repeat on the other side.

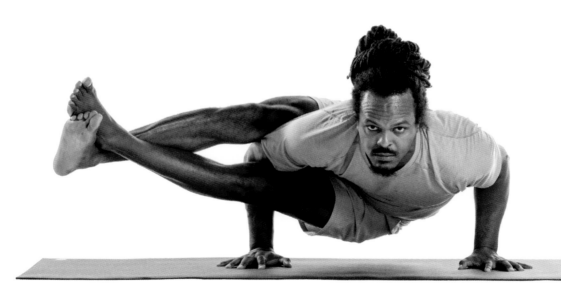

SHALABHASANA A AND B
(shah-lah-BAHS-anna)

shalabh = grasshopper, locust   asana = pose

LOCUST POSE

First drishti: nasikagra—tip of the nose

1. From chaturanga dandasana (page 54), on an exhale, lower to the ground with the legs straight. Place the arms by your side, with the palms facing upward.

2. On an inhale, lift the feet, head, and chest from the mat, keeping the legs and ankles together. Press the backs of the hands down into the mat. Engage the core to support the lower back. Keep the bottom ribs and the front of the hips pressing into the ground even as you lift the feet, head, and chest. This is shalabhasana A (see figure a).

3. Draw the navel into the spine to engage uddiyana bandha, stabilize the core, and bring the breath into the rib cage. Engage the inner thighs toward the midline to lift the pelvic floor and engage mula bandha. Maintain the soft sound of the breath through the contraction of the throat to gently apply jalandhara bandha.

4. Hold for as long as needed.

5. Maintain the lift in the legs and chest and then bring the hands to the mat, palms down, next to the lowest ribs. Press the hands into the mat but keep the elbows bent and the work in the back. This is shalabhasana B (see figure b).

6. Draw the navel into the spine to engage uddiyana bandha, stabilize the core, and bring the breath into the rib cage. Engage the inner thighs toward the midline to lift the pelvic floor and engage mula bandha. Maintain the soft sound of the breath through the contraction of the throat to gently apply jalandhara bandha.

7. Hold for as long as needed.

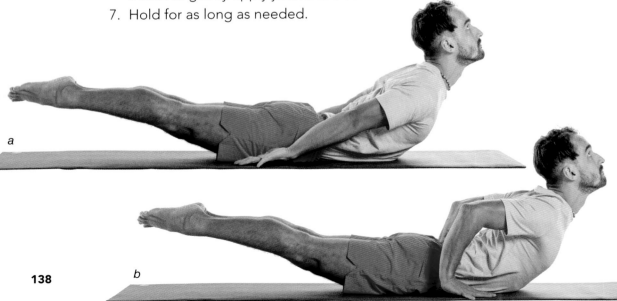

a

b

SHALABHASANA VARIATION

(*shah-lah-BAHS-anna*)

shalabh = grasshopper, locust   asana = pose

LOCUST POSE

First drishti: nasikagra—tip of the nose

1. From shalabhasana B (page 138), on an inhale, bring the arms straight in front of the shoulders, and turn the palms to face the floor. Engage the core to support the lower back. Keep the bottom ribs and the front of the hips pressing into the ground even as you lift the feet, head, and chest.

2. Draw the navel into the spine to engage uddiyana bandha, stabilize the core, and bring the breath into the rib cage. Engage the inner thighs toward the midline to lift the pelvic floor and engage mula bandha. Maintain the soft sound of the breath through the contraction of the throat to gently apply jalandhara bandha.

3. Hold for as long as needed.

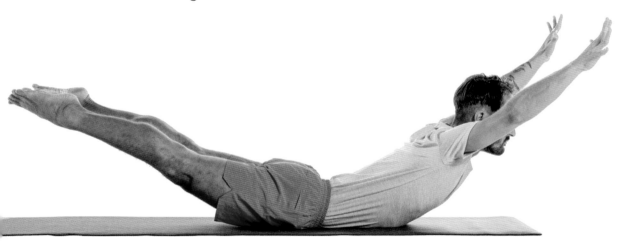

BHEKASANA
(beh-KAHS-ahna)
bheka = frog   asana = pose

FROG POSE

First drishti: nasikagra—tip of the nose

1. From chaturanga dandasana (page 54), lower the entire body to the ground on an exhale.

2. Bend the knees to bring the heels toward the sitz bones. Reach the arms back and catch the ankles from the inside. As you press the feet toward the ground outside of the hips, spin the palms over the tops of the feet, allowing the fingers to point in the same direction as the toes. The elbows stack on top of the wrists to apply downward pressure on the feet while you simultaneously lift the chest.

3. Draw the navel into the spine to engage uddiyana bandha, stabilize the core, and bring the breath into the rib cage. Engage the inner thighs toward the midline to lift the pelvic floor and engage mula bandha. Maintain the soft sound of the breath through the contraction of the throat to gently apply jalandhara bandha.

4. Hold for as long as needed.

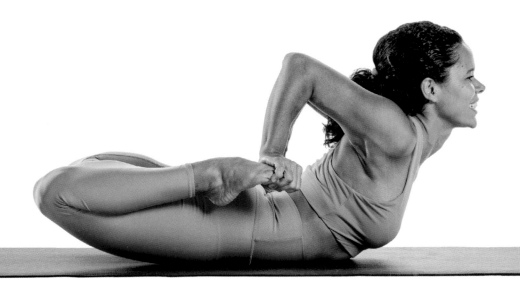

SUPTA VIRASANA

(SOUP-tah veer-AHS-anna)

supta = reclining   vira = hero   asana = pose

RECLINING HERO POSE

First drishti: nasikagra—tip of the nose

1. From adho mukha svanasana (page 56), on an inhale, lower the knees to the ground to come to a kneeling position. Sit the hips between the feet, with the toes pointing directly behind.

2. On an exhale, lean back and place the elbows on the mat for support. Continue to lower until you are lying flat on your back.

3. Draw the navel into the spine to engage uddiyana bandha, stabilize the core, and bring the breath into the rib cage. Engage the inner thighs toward the midline to lift the pelvic floor and engage mula bandha. Maintain the soft sound of the breath through the contraction of the throat to gently apply jalandhara bandha.

4. Hold for as long as needed.

Modifications

- To ease the stretch in the quadriceps, do not recline fully.
- To ease the tension in the knees, sit on a block and do not recline.

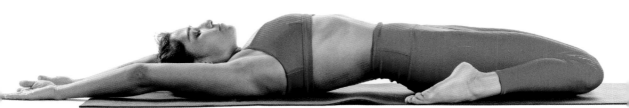

BALASANA

(bahl-AHS-anna)

bala = child   asana = pose

CHILD'S POSE

Drishti: none, eyes closed

1. From supta virasana (page 141), on an inhale, return to a seated position with the hips between the heels. Use the elbows and hands as you come up to keep the spine centered and avoid tilting to the side.

2. On an exhale, fold forward, resting the forehead on the ground. The arms can reach forward or can rest by the hips. Bring the big toes to touch in the center, and allow the hips and lower back to relax.

3. Rest here for as long as needed.

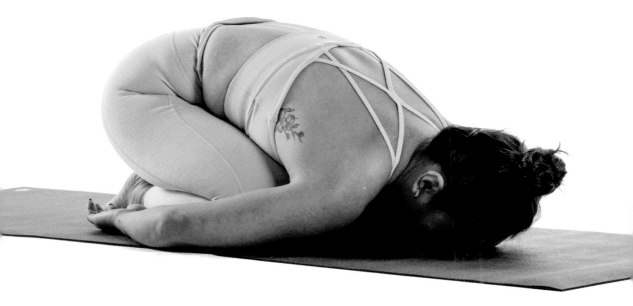

DHANURASANA

(dahn-you-RAHS-anna)

danura = wheel   asana = pose

WHEEL POSE

BOW POSE

First drishti: nasikagra—tip of the nose

1. From chaturanga dandasana (page 54), on an exhale, lower to the ground with the legs straight. Bend the knees, reach the arms back, and grab the ankles from the outside so that the thumbs point downward.

2. On an inhale, lift the feet, head, and chest, creating opposition between the hands and the feet to help lift the upper chest and thighs higher off the ground. Keep the bottom ribs and the front of the hips pressing into the ground even as you lift the feet, head, and chest.

3. Draw the navel into the spine to engage uddiyana bandha, stabilize the core, and bring the breath into the rib cage. Engage the inner thighs toward the midline to lift the pelvic floor and engage mula bandha. Maintain the soft sound of the breath through the contraction of the throat to gently apply jalandhara bandha.

4. Hold for as long as needed.

Modification

To ease tension in the front of the shoulders, use a strap to reach the feet or ankles. You can also do one side at a time, with or without a strap.

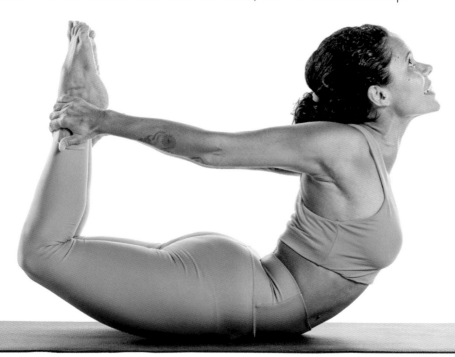

PARSVA DHANURASANA

(PARS-vah dahn-you-RAHS-anna)

parsva = side   danura = wheel   asana = pose

FALLEN WHEEL POSE

SIDE BOW POSE

First drishti: nasikagra—tip of the nose

1. From dhanurasana (page 143), on an exhale, remain mindful of the shape of the body in dhanurasana, and roll to the right side. Do not let the head touch the ground, and keep the right-side ribs touching the ground.
2. Let the shoulder roll completely under the body to stretch the front of the chest. Keep the toes touching and hips reaching forward.
3. Draw the navel into the spine to engage uddiyana bandha, stabilize the core, and bring the breath into the rib cage. Engage the inner thighs toward the midline to lift the pelvic floor and engage mula bandha. Maintain the soft sound of the breath through the contraction of the throat to gently apply jalandhara bandha.
4. Hold for as long as needed, then repeat on the other side.

Modification

To ease tension in the front of the shoulders, use a strap to reach the feet or ankles.

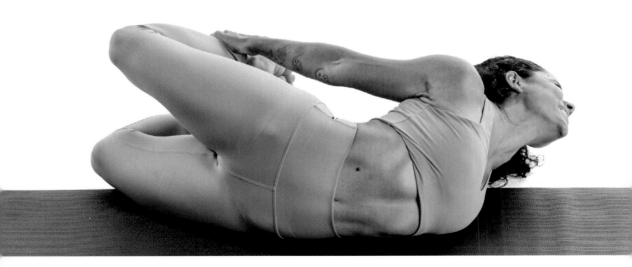

RAJA KAPOTASANA

(RAH-jah kah-po-TAHS-anna)

raja = king   kapota = pigeon   asana = pose

KING PIGEON POSE

First drishti: nasikagra—tip of the nose

1. From dhanurasana (page 143), on an exhale, place both hands on the floor, shoulder-width apart and fingers pointing forward. Keep the knees bent.
2. On an inhale, straighten both arms, drawing the shoulder blades down the back.
3. On an exhale, reach the crown of the head toward the toes as the knees bend, and draw the feet toward the head.
4. Draw the navel into the spine to engage uddiyana bandha, stabilize the core, and bring the breath into the rib cage. Engage the inner thighs toward the midline to lift the pelvic floor and engage mula bandha. Maintain the soft sound of the breath through the contraction of the throat to gently apply jalandhara bandha.
5. Hold for as long as needed.

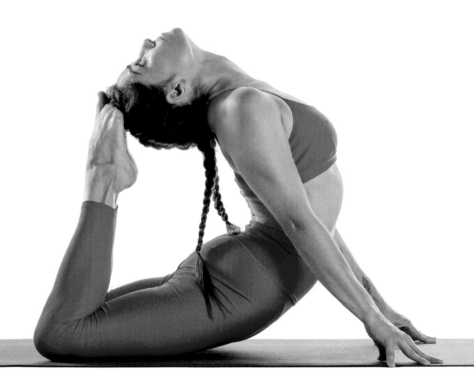

USTRASANA
(oos-TRAHS-anna)
ustra = camel   asana = pose

CAMEL POSE

First drishti: nasikagra—tip of the nose

1. From adho mukha svanasana (page 56), on an inhale, bring both knees to the ground, hip-width apart and shins parallel. Bring the torso upright, and bring both hands to the waist.

2. On an exhale, extend from the base of the spine and lean back, keeping the hips over the knees and continuing to press the hips forward. Reach the hands down to hold the heels. Internally rotate the thighs, continuing to lift the chest. Allow the head to drop back.

3. Draw the navel into the spine to engage uddiyana bandha, stabilize the core, and bring the breath into the rib cage. Engage the inner thighs toward the midline to lift the pelvic floor and engage mula bandha. Maintain the soft sound of the breath through the contraction of the throat to gently apply jalandhara bandha.

4. Hold for as long as needed.

Modification

To decrease the backbend, place blocks outside of the heels and reach the hands to the blocks instead of the heels.

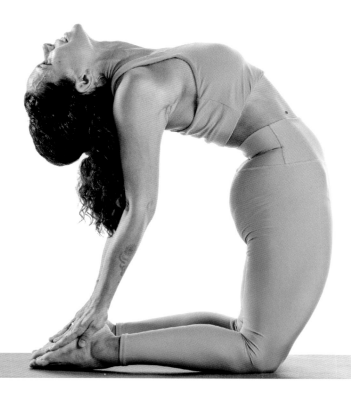

LAGHU VAJRASANA

(LAH-goo vaj-RAHS-ahna)

laghu = little   vajra = thunderbolt   asana = pose

LITTLE THUNDERBOLT POSE

First drishti: nasikagra—tip of the nose

1. From adho mukha svanasana (page 56), on an inhale, jump the knees between the hands and come to a kneeling position at the top of the mat with the hands on the hips.
2. On an exhale, place the hands on the ankles with the fingers to the outside and the thumbs to the inside of the ankle, then lean back and lower the crown of the head to the mat behind the feet, keeping the hips pressing forward and the back in extension.
3. Hold here for five breaths.
4. On an inhale, press into the hands and lift the body back to the starting position, kneeling with the hands on the hips.

Modification

If your knees lift as you recline into the pose or you cannot return to the starting position, place a block where your head would touch the ground and only lower to that point until you have built enough strength to lower the crown of the head to the ground.

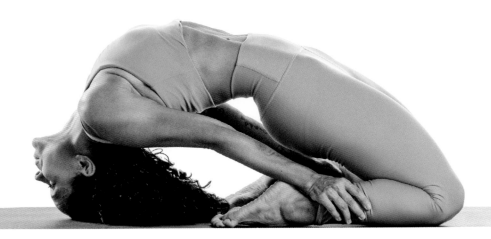

KAPOTASANA A AND B

(kah-po-TAHS-anna)

kapota = pigeon   asana = pose

PIGEON POSE

First drishti: nasikagra—tip of the nose

1. From adho mukha svanasana (page 56), on an inhale, bring both knees to the ground, hip-width apart and shins parallel. Bring the palms together to the prayer position.

2. On an exhale, extend from the base of the spine and lean back, keeping the hips over the knees and continuing to press the hips forward. Reach the hands behind, stretching across the front of the body. Keep extending the spine until the hands touch the ground.

3. Internally rotate the thighs and keep lifting and expanding the chest. Keeping the external rotation of the upper arm, walk the hands toward the feet until they can grab the heels.

4. On an inhale, straighten the arms as much as possible, lengthening the spine, and then on an exhale, rest the elbows on the ground, drawing them toward the centerline. This is kapotasana A (see figure *a*).

5. Draw the navel into the spine to engage uddiyana bandha, stabilize the core, and bring the breath into the rib cage. Engage the inner thighs toward the midline to lift the pelvic floor and engage mula bandha. Maintain the soft sound of the breath through the contraction of the throat to gently apply jalandhara bandha.

6. Hold for as long as needed.

7. Release the hands from the heels and place the palms on the ground just outside of the feet, fingers pointing toward the front of the mat (see figure *b*). On an inhale, straighten the arms and look toward the feet. This is kapotasana B.

8. Draw the navel into the spine to engage uddiyana bandha, stabilize the core, and bring the breath into the rib cage. Engage the inner thighs toward the midline to lift the pelvic floor and engage mula bandha. Maintain the soft sound of the breath through the contraction of the throat to gently apply jalandhara bandha.

9. Hold for as long as needed.

Modification

If this is too difficult, use camel pose (page 146).

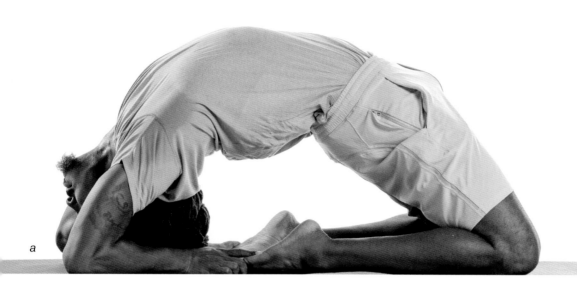

a

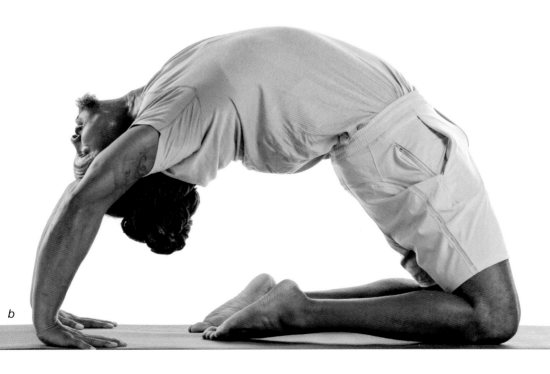

b

SUPTA VAJRASANA

(SOOP-tah vaj-RAHS-ahna)

supta = reclined   vajra = thunderbolt   asana = pose

RECLINED THUNDERBOLT POSE

First drishti: nasikagra—tip of the nose

1. This pose is typically practiced with a partner who sits in front of you, places their legs on top of your knees for stability and holds on to your wrists to help maintain the connection to the feet during the entire movement.

2. From adho mukha svanasana (page 56), on an inhale, jump through the hands to a seated position, with the hips between the hands and the legs extended straight out front. Fold the legs into a full lotus position, bringing the right foot in first, followed by the left foot.

3. Reach the arms behind the back to hold the same side foot (i.e., right hand holds the right foot; left hand holds the left foot) (see figure *a*). Tightly hold the feet in this position.

4. On an exhale, lean back, find an extension of the spine, and touch the crown of the head to the ground (see figure *b*). Hold for five breaths and then on an inhale, return to an upright seat.

5. On an exhale, perform the movement again, this time immediately returning on the inhale. Repeat two more times, then repeat step 3 once again, holding at the bottom for five breaths.

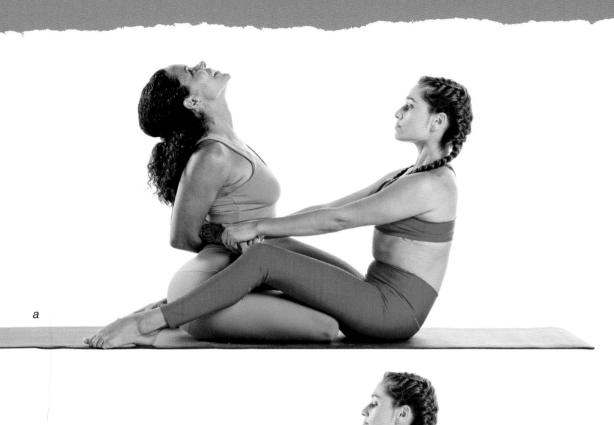

a

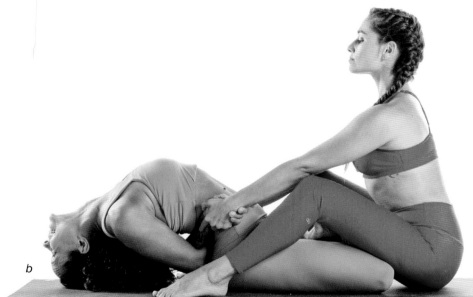

b

BAKASANA B
(bahk-AHS-anna)
baka = crane   asana = pose

CRANE POSE

First drishti: nasikagra—tip of the nose

1. From adho mukha svanasana (page 56), bend the knees generously and then jump directly into bakasana A (page 60), bringing the knees to the triceps and pressing down into the hands to straighten the arms (see figures *a-c*).
2. Draw the navel into the spine to engage uddiyana bandha. Lift the pelvic floor to engage mula bandha.
3. Hold for as long as needed.

Modification

Jumping directly into bakasana A takes courage and strength. You can place a pillow on the ground in front of your head if you are scared of falling forward. You can also start from a closer position by walking your feet closer to your hands before jumping.

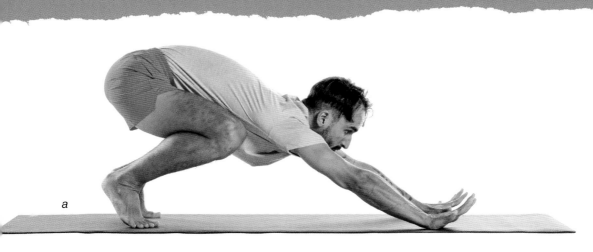

a

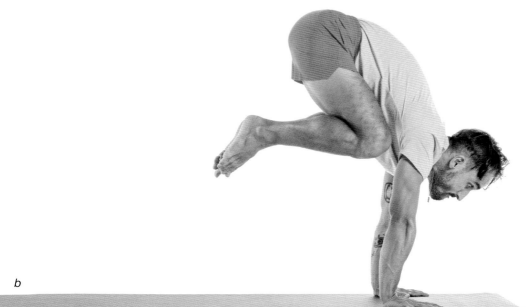

b

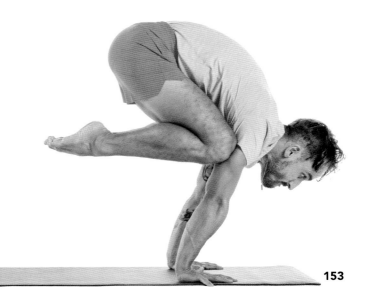

c

153

ADHO MUKHA VRKSASANA

(AH-doh MOO-kah vree-KAHS-anna)

adho = downward   mukha = facing   vrka = tree   asana = pose

HANDSTAND

Drishti: Floor between hands

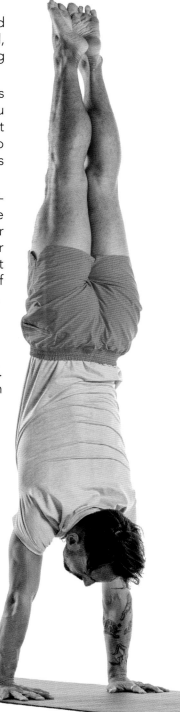

1. From samasthiti (page 51), on an exhale, fold forward and place the hands flat on the ground, shoulder-width apart with the fingers facing forward.

2. On an inhale, shift your weight to your hands and lift the legs to a full vertical position. You can do this by either kicking one leg up at a time, jumping into a tuck, or pressing up through a pike or a straddle. Use the fingertips to control the balance.

3. Draw the navel into the spine to engage uddi-yana bandha, stabilize the core, and bring the breath into the rib cage. Engage the inner thighs toward the midline to lift the pelvic floor and engage mula bandha. Maintain the soft sound of the breath through the contraction of the throat to gently apply jalandhara bandha.

4. Hold for as long as needed.

Modification

To help with balance, start by practicing against a wall. As you gain strength, stamina, and balance, you can move away from the wall.

BHARADVAJASANA

(bah-rahd-vah-JAHS-anna)

Bharadvaj = the sage named Bharadvaj   asana = pose

SAGE BHARADVAJA'S POSE

Sixth drishti: parsva—to the right

Seventh drishti: parsva—to the left

1. From adho mukha svanasana (page 56), on an inhale, jump through the hands to a seated position, with the hips between the hands. Extend the right leg straight out front, and bend the left leg with the left foot outside of the hip and the toes pointing to the back.

2. On an exhale, place the right foot in a half lotus position on top of the left thigh. Reach the right arm behind the back to grab the right toes with the right hand. Place the left hand under the right knee with the palm facing down and the fingers under the knee. Keep both sitz bones anchored as best you can, allowing the twist to start from the base of the spine and extend all the way up through the neck.

3. Draw the navel into the spine to engage uddiyana bandha, stabilize the core, and bring the breath into the rib cage. Lift the pelvic floor and engage mula bandha. Maintain the soft sound of the breath through the contraction of the throat to gently apply jalandhara bandha.

4. Hold for as long as needed, then repeat on the other side.

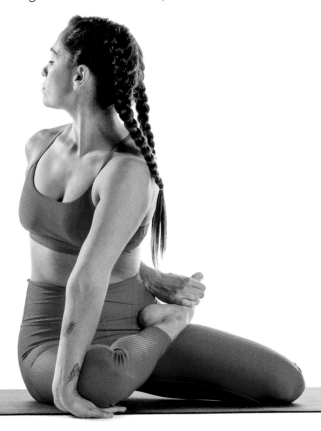

ARDHA MATSYENDRASANA

(ARD-ha maht-syen-DRAHS-anna)

ardha = half   matsyendra = lord of the fishes   asana = pose

HALF LORD OF THE FISH POSE

Drishti: Gaze to the side

1. From adho mukha svanasana (page 56), on an inhale, jump through the hands to a seated position. Bend the right knee toward the sky, and cross the right foot to the outside of the left knee. Bend the left leg, and bring the left foot to the outside of the right hip.

2. On an exhale, twist toward the right side, placing the left elbow outside of the right knee. Wrap the left arm down the right leg, and reach the left hand to the inside of the right foot for a bind. Reach the right arm behind the back, and slide the right hand into the left hip pocket. Keep both sitz bones anchored as best you can, allowing the twist to start from the base of the spine and extend all the way up through the neck.

3. Draw the navel into the spine to engage uddiyana bandha, stabilize the core, and bring the breath into the rib cage. Engage the inner thighs toward the midline to lift the pelvic floor and engage mula bandha. Maintain the soft sound of the breath through the contraction of the throat to gently apply jalandhara bandha.

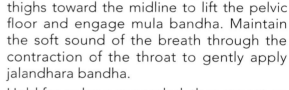

4. Hold for as long as needed, then repeat on the other side.

Modification

If this is too difficult, use marichyasana C (page 105).

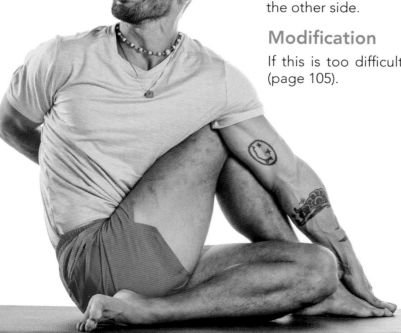

ADHO MUKHA KAPOTASANA

(AH-doh MOO-kah kah-po-TAHS-anna)

adho = downward   mukha = face
kapota = pigeon   asana = pose

DOWNWARD-FACING PIGEON POSE

First drishti: nasikagra—tip of the nose

1. From adho mukha svanasana (page 56), on an inhale, lift the right leg behind you. On an exhale, swing the leg forward, bringing the right knee behind the right wrist, and sit with the legs in this position. Rotate the right leg to the right, with the right shin parallel to the top edge of the mat. Extend the left leg directly behind the left hip, with the top of the left thigh resting on the ground.

2. On an inhale, extend the spine and straighten the arms.

3. On an exhale, fold forward over the right shin, bringing the forehead to rest on the ground and reaching both arms forward. Keep both hips squared with the front of the mat by pressing the front of the left hip strongly into the ground.

4. Hold for as long as needed, then repeat on the other side.

Modification

To ease the stretch, do not fold forward.

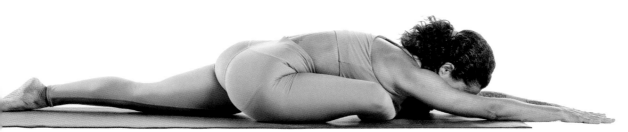

EKA PADA RAJA KAPOTASANA

(e-kah pah-dah rah-jah kah-po-TAHS-anna)

eka = one pada = foot raja = king
kapota = pigeon asana = pose

ONE-LEG KING PIGEON POSE

First drishti: nasikagra—tip of the nose

1. From adho mukha kapotasana (page 157), sit up and place the hands on the mat in front of the right shin, shoulder-width apart.
2. On an inhale, press the hands into the mat and lift the torso, looking up toward the sky.
3. On an exhale, while maintaining the alignment of the hips, bend the left knee toward the head. Reach the left hand back to clasp the inside of the left foot. Continue to bend the back leg while the crown of the head reaches toward the back foot. Reach the right hand back, clasping the outside edge of the left foot with the right hand as well.
4. Draw the navel into the spine to engage uddiyana bandha, stabilize the core, and bring the breath into the rib cage. Engage the inner thighs toward the midline to lift the pelvic floor, ground the hips, and engage mula bandha. Maintain the soft sound of the breath through the contraction of the throat to gently apply jalandhara bandha.
5. Hold for as long as needed, then repeat on the other side.

Modification

If this is too difficult, use adho mukha kapotasana (page 157).

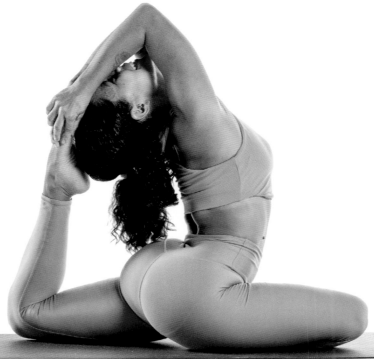

GOMUKHASANA

(goh-mook-AHS-anna)

go = cow   mukha = face   asana = pose

COW FACE POSE

First drishti: nasikagra—tip of the nose

1. From adho mukha svanasana (page 56), on an inhale, lift the left leg behind you. On an exhale, swing the leg forward, bringing the left knee behind the left wrist, and sit with the legs in this position.

2. Lean toward the left side, then swing the right leg around to the front, bending the knee to stack it on top of the left knee, right thigh over the left thigh, then sitting the hips between the feet.

3. On an inhale, sit up, lengthen the spine, and lift the chin. Raise the left arm, bending the left elbow so it points toward the sky, and the left hand reaches down the back. Bend the right elbow so it points downward, reach the hand behind the back, and clasp both hands together (see figure a).

4. On an exhale, fold forward over the knees, leading with the chest (see figure b).

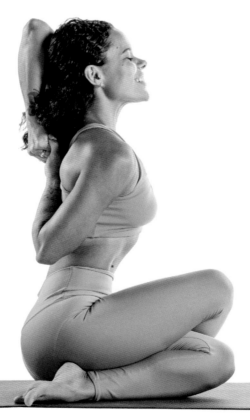

a

(continued)

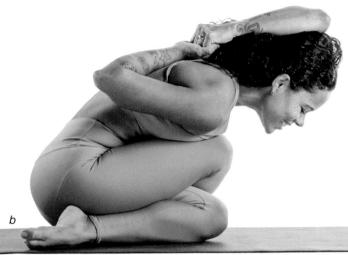

b

5. Draw the navel into the spine to engage uddiyana bandha, stabilize the core, and bring the breath into the rib cage. Engage the inner thighs toward the midline to lift the pelvic floor and engage mula bandha. Maintain the soft sound of the breath through the contraction of the throat to gently apply jalandhara bandha.

6. Hold for as long as needed, then repeat on the other side.

Modifications

- To ease the stretch, do not fold forward.
- To ease shoulder tension, use a strap to bridge the distance between the hands.
- To perform the classical ashtanga version of this pose, do not allow the shins to separate and the hips to sit on the ground. Bring the shins as close to parallel as possible, balancing completely on one shin and using the top of the other foot for stability. The arms mirror the legs in this version—if the right thigh is on top, the right elbow reaches up to the ceiling. Fold forward, maintain the same engagement in the bandhas, and hold for as long as needed before repeating on the other side (see figure).

SUPTA URDHVA PADA VAJRASANA

(*SOOP-tah OORD-vah PAH-dah vaj-RAHS-ahna*)

supta = reclined   urdhva = upward
pada = foot   vajra = thunderbolt   asana = pose

SLEEPING UPWARD LIFTING LEG THUNDERBOLT POSE

First drishti: nasikagra—tip of the nose

1. From adho mukha svanasana (p. 56), on an inhale, jump through the hands to a seated position with the hips between the hands and the legs extended straight out front, and then on an exhale, lie down on your back.

2. On an inhale, bring your feet, legs, and hips over your shoulders and let the feet rest on the floor behind the crown of your head, similar to halasana (page 184).

3. On an exhale, bring the right foot to a half lotus while reaching the right arm across the lower back, grabbing the toes of the right foot with the right hand. Hold on to the big toe of the left foot with the first and second fingers of the left hand. Keep the left leg extended (see figure *a*).

4. On an inhale, roll up to a seated position and bend the left knee, bringing the left foot outside of the hip to twist with the half lotus, similar to bharadvajasana (page 155) (see figure *b*).

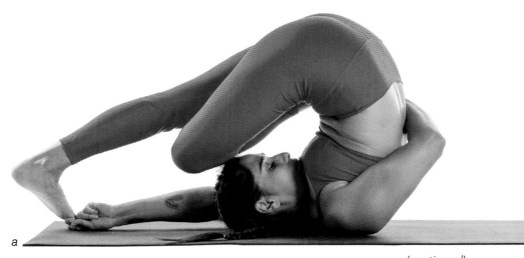

a

(continued)

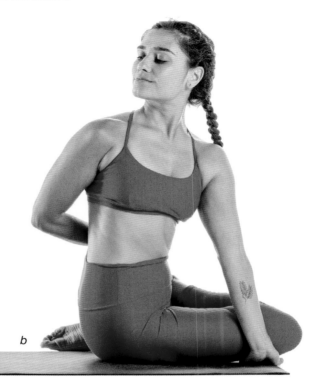

b

5. Draw the navel into the spine to engage uddiyana bandha, stabilize the core, and bring the breath into the rib cage. Lift the pelvic floor to engage mula bandha and relax the hip muscles. Maintain the soft sound of the breath through the contraction of the throat to gently apply jalandhara bandha.

6. Hold for as long as needed, then repeat on the other side.

EKA PADA SIRSASANA

(*e-kah pah-dah sheer-SHAHS-anna*)

eka = one   pada = foot   sirsa = head   asana = pose

ONE FOOT TO HEAD POSTURE

First drishti: nasikagra—tip of the nose

1. From adho mukha svanasana (page 56), on an inhale, jump through the hands to a seated position with the hips between the hands and the legs extended straight out front.
2. On an exhale, bring the right shin behind the neck. Pay attention to the rotation in the right hip, allowing the lower leg to move completely down the back of the neck toward the shoulders (see figure *a*).
3. Fold forward and keep the head pressing back on the leg so the spine remains as straight as possible (see figure *b*).
4. Draw the navel into the spine to engage uddiyana bandha, stabilize the core, and bring the breath into the rib cage. Lift the pelvic floor to engage mula bandha and relax the hip muscles. Maintain the soft sound of the breath through the contraction of the throat to gently apply jalandhara bandha.
5. Hold for as long as needed, then repeat on the other side.

Modification

If this is too difficult, use downward-facing pigeon pose (page 157).

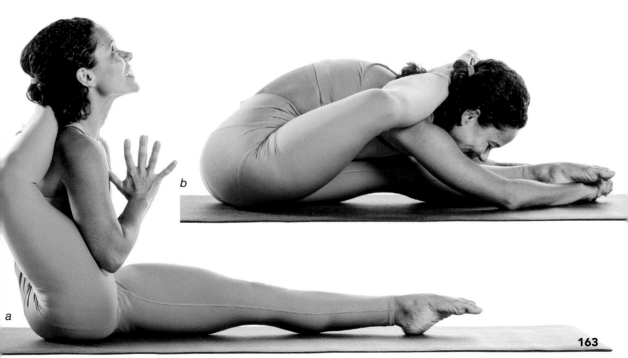

a

b

DWI PADA SIRSASANA

(*dwee pah-dah sheer-SHAHS-ahna*)

dwi = two   pada = foot   sirsa = head   asana = pose

FEET BEHIND THE HEAD POSE

First drishti: nasikagra—tip of the nose

1. From adho mukha svanasana (p. 56), on an inhale, jump through the hands to a seated position with the hips between the hands and the legs extended straight out front.

2. Bring the left leg behind the head, allowing the shin of the left leg to rest behind the neck. Lift the chest and head up to counteract the pressure from the leg. Engage the hamstrings of the left leg to stabilize and hold the leg in place.

3. Bring the right leg behind the head as well, placing it behind the left leg and crossing the feet at the ankles. Stay balanced on your sitz bones.

4. Bring the hands to heart center, pressing the palms together.

5. Draw the navel into the spine to engage uddiyana bandha, stabilize the core, and bring the breath into the rib cage. Lift the pelvic floor to engage mula bandha and relax the hip muscles. Maintain the soft sound of the breath through the contraction of the throat to gently apply jalandhara bandha.

6. Hold for five breaths.

7. To release the pose, press the hands down into the ground, about shoulder-width apart, lifting the hips off the ground. Uncross the ankles, extending the legs forward and straightening both the arms and legs into titibhasana A (page 166). Move the legs through bakasana (page 60) and jump back in chaturanga dandasana (page 54).

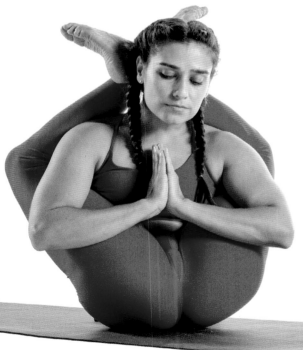

YOGA NIDRASANA
(YOH-gah nee-DRAHS-ahna)
yoga = unite   nidra = sleep   asana = pose

SLEEPING YOGI POSE

First drishti: nasikagra—tip of the nose

1. From adho mukha svanasana (p. 56), on an inhale, jump through the hands to a seated position with the hips between the hands and the legs extended straight out front. Lie down on your back.

2. Bring the left leg behind the head, allowing the shin of the left leg to rest behind the neck. Lift the chest and head up to counteract the pressure from the leg. Engage the hamstrings of the left leg to stabilize and hold the leg in place.

3. Bring the right leg behind the head as well, placing it behind the left leg and crossing the feet at the ankles.

4. Bring the hands behind the lower back and clasp the hands together in a bind.

5. Draw the navel into the spine to engage uddiyana bandha, stabilize the core, and bring the breath into the rib cage. Lift the pelvic floor to engage mula bandha and relax the hip muscles. Maintain the soft sound of the breath through the contraction of the throat to gently apply jalandhara bandha.

6. Hold for five breaths.

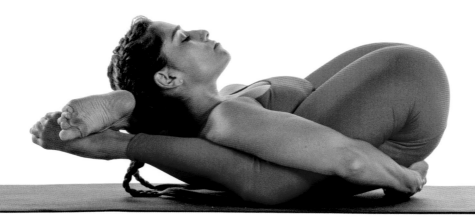

TITIBHASANA A, B, C, AND D
(tee-tee-BAHS-ahna)
titibha = fly, insect   asana = pose

FIREFLY POSE

First drishti: nasikagra—tip of the nose

1. From adho mukha svanasana (p. 56), on an inhale, jump the feet to the outside of the hands at the top of the mat.
2. On an exhale, brace the shoulders behind the knees and bring both hands to the ground, shoulder-width apart.
3. On an inhale, lift and straighten the legs forward while balancing on your hands. Point your toes and actively engage the inner thighs. This is titibhasana A (see figure *a*). After a few rounds of breath, release the feet to the floor.
4. On an inhale, stand up onto the feet as you retain the position of the shoulders behind the back of the knees and thighs. Bring the arms behind the back and bind the hands by clasping them together. Look through your legs and gaze up at the sky. This is titibhasana B (see figure *b*). Hold for a few breaths.
5. Maintaining the bind of the hands behind the back, walk forward five steps and backward for five steps, taking your time and breathing as you walk. This is titibhasana C (see figure *c*).
6. Bring the feet as close together as you can, pushing the shoulders farther behind the legs. Heels touch together and the toes are allowed to turn out for balance. Bring the hands to bind behind the head. This is titibhasana D (see figure *d*).
7. To exit this pose, plant the hands on the ground shoulder-width apart and move through titibhasana A before jumping back through bakasana (page 60) to chaturanga dandasana (page 54).

Modification

If the hands don't touch behind the back, use a towel or strap to connect the hands.

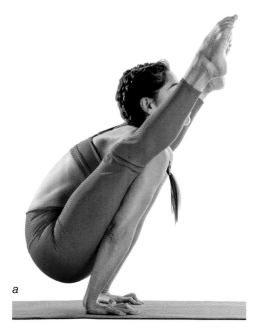

a

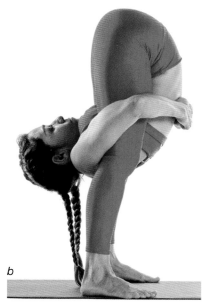

b

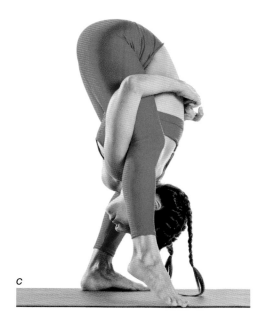

c

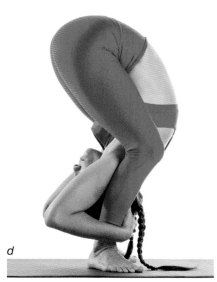

d

KARANDAVASANA

(kah-rahn-dah-VAHS-ahna)

karandava = Himalayan goose   asana = pose

DUCK POSE

First drishti: nasikagra—tip of the nose

1. From adho mukha svanasana (p. 56), on an inhale, lower both elbows to the ground, keeping the forearms parallel.

2. On an exhale, walk the feet in closer to the arms to lift the hips.

3. On an inhale, lift by transferring the weight of the body over the shoulders and balance the hips and legs in the air, coming into pincha mayurasana (page 67).

4. On an exhale, bring the legs into a full lotus position with the right leg positioned first to the top of the left thigh. The left leg completes the lotus by crossing the foot to the right thigh (see figure a).

5. On an exhale, fold the lotus in toward the chest, bringing the knees down on the back of the upper arms (see figure b). Hold here for five breaths.

6. On an inhale, lift back up in the same manner coming into pincha mayurasana before releasing completely out of the pose.

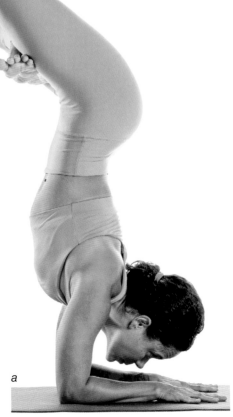

a

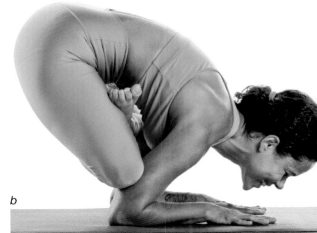

b

MAYURASANA

(mah-yoor-AHS-ahna)

mayura = peacock   asana = pose

PEACOCK POSE

First drishti: nasikagra—tip of the nose

1. From adho mukha svanasana (page 56), on an inhale, hop forward to your knees and sit on top of the feet with the knees open wide.
2. On an exhale, place the hands on the floor with the heels of the hands touching, fingers turned backward and the elbows positioned into the belly/diaphragm area.
3. On an inhale, lean the weight of the body forward onto the elbows, lifting the entire body to balance on the back of the elbows. Extend the legs straight back.
4. Stay for as long as needed.

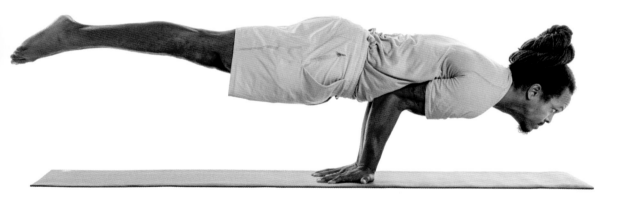

NAKRASANA

(*nah-KRAHS-anna*)

nakra = crocodile   asana = pose

CROCODILE POSE

First drishti: nasikagra—tip of the nose

1. From adho mukha svanasana (page 56), on an inhale, shift the shoulders forward and come to a high plank position.
2. On an exhale, lower into chaturanga dandasana (page 54), holding the body in a straight line (see figure *a*).
3. On an inhale, jump all four limbs off the ground, and move forward a few inches (see figure *b*). Exhale to land softly back into chaturanga dandasana.
4. While the body is lifted off the floor, maintain a horizontal position. Bend the elbows in toward the ribs, and pull the hands by the chest to keep the shape of a crocodile with short arms. Anticipate the landing, and reach out to the floor slowly to soften the landing by applying pressure with the hands as you bend the elbows. Work with a bouncing feeling to minimize the shock of the posture.
5. Repeat this action three times forward and three times backward.

Modification

To build strength for this pose, hold a high plank for 10 breaths, then hold a low plank (chaturanga) for 10 breaths. Repeat.

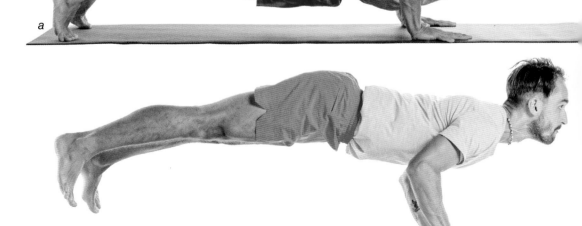

a

b

VATAYANASANA
(vah-ta-yah-NAHS-ahna)
vatayana = horse   asana = pose

HORSE FACE POSE

First drishti: nasikagra—tip of the nose

1. From samasthiti (page 51), on an inhale, bring the right leg into a half lotus with the right foot on top of the thigh, reaching the right arm behind the back to hold the right foot. On an exhale, fold forward.

2. On an inhale look up halfway, lengthening your spine.

3. On an exhale, plant both hands at the top of the mat, shoulder-width apart, and jump back to a push-up position while maintaining the half lotus position in the right leg.

4. On an inhale, press the arms straight to the upward-facing dog position and keep the hips, thighs, and knees off the ground. Maintain the half lotus position in the right leg.

5. On an exhale, press back into adho mukha svanasana (page 56) with the right leg in half lotus.

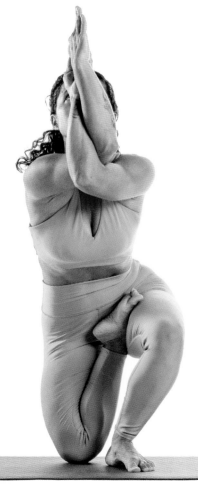

(continued)

6. On an inhale, jump the left foot forward to the hands, then turn the foot out, externally rotating the leg so the left knee bends over the foot in the same direction. Bring the right knee down directly behind the left heel and then lift your torso upward into the upright posture. Your foundation here is the left foot and the right knee.

7. Wrap the left arm under the right arm and spiral the forearms, bringing the palms to touch and pointing the fingers up to the ceiling. The fingers will not be in line here; the left fingers will come to the palm of the right hand.

8. Draw the navel into the spine to engage uddiyana bandha, stabilize the core, and bring the breath into the rib cage. Lift the pelvic floor to engage mula bandha and relax the hip muscles. Maintain the soft sound of the breath through the contraction of the throat to gently apply jalandhara bandha.

9. Stay here for five breaths.

10. Release from this pose the same way you entered it, keeping the right leg in the half lotus position through chaturanga dandasana (page 54), urdhva mukha svanasana (page 55), adho mukha svanasana (page 56), ardha uttanasana (page 72), uttanasana (page 70), and urdhva hastasana (page 52). Release the right leg from the half lotus position when you are standing back at the top of the mat.

11. Repeat on the other side.

PARIGHASANA

(pah-ree-GAHS-ahna)

parigha = gate   asana = pose

GATE POSE

Ninth drishti: urdhva or antara—up to the sky

1. From adho mukha svanasana (page 56), on an inhale, jump through the hands to a seated position with the hips between the hands and the legs extended straight out front. Bend the right knee, placing the right foot outside of the right hip and bringing the right knee to point out to the right side.

2. On an exhale, reach the right arm over the head and toward the left foot, side stretching toward the extended leg with the left shoulder coming inside the left leg for extra leverage to open the right side body.

3. Draw the navel into the spine to engage uddiyana bandha, stabilize the core, and bring the breath into the rib cage. Lift the pelvic floor to engage mula bandha and relax the hip muscles. Maintain the soft sound of the breath through the contraction of the throat to gently apply jalandhara bandha.

4. Stay for as long as needed, then repeat on the other side.

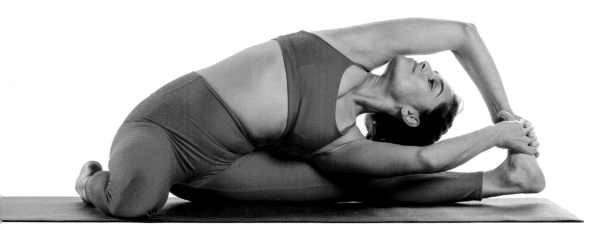

MUKTA HASTA SIRSASANA A

(MOOK-tah HAHS-tah sheer-SHAHS-anna)

mukta = liberated hasta = hand sirsa = head asana = pose

TRIPOD HEADSTAND

First drishti: nasikagra—tip of the nose

1. From balasana (page 142), on an inhale, place your palms on the floor, shoulder-width apart with the fingers pointing forward. Place the top of the head between the hands and about six inches (15 cm) behind, ensuring that you can see your hands. The elbows should form 90-degree angles. The top of the head and the two hands form the tripod foundation for this inversion.

2. On an exhale, lift the knees off the ground and shift the weight to the head. Tip toe the feet in as close as possible, keeping both legs straight until the hips are over the shoulders.

3. In an inhale, lift both legs together or lift one leg and then the other, to come into a full inversion. The body is in a straight line, with weight on both hands and the top of the head (see figure a).

4. Draw the navel into the spine to engage uddiyana bandha, stabilize the core, and bring the breath into the rib cage. Engage the inner thighs toward the midline to lift the pelvic floor and engage mula bandha. Maintain the soft sound of the breath through the contraction of the throat to gently apply jalandhara bandha.

5. Hold for as long as needed.

Modification

To work on balance, after creating the foundation, bring each knee on top of each elbow and bring the feet together in the center (see figure b). Stay here.

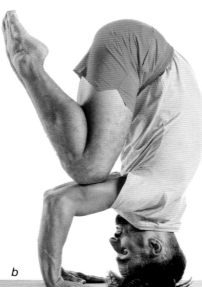

a

b

MUKTA HASTA SIRSASANA B

(MOOK-tah HAHS-tah sheer-SHAHS-anna)

mukta = liberated   hasta = hand   sirsa = head   asana = pose

TRIPOD HEADSTAND

First drishti: nasikagra—tip of the nose

1. From balasana (page 142), on an inhale, place your palms on the floor, shoulder-width apart with the fingers pointing forward. Place the top of the head between the hands. Extend the arms forward shoulder-width apart and turn the palms upward toward the ceiling. Press through the back of your hands to stabilize the shoulder girdle.

2. On an exhale, lift the knees off the ground and shift the weight to the head. Tip toe the feet in as close as possible, keeping both legs straight until the hips are over the shoulders.

3. On an inhale, lift both legs together or lift one leg and then the other, to come into a full inversion. The body is in a straight line, with weight on the back of both hands and the top of the head.

4. Draw the navel into the spine to engage uddiyana bandha, stabilize the core, and bring the breath into the rib cage. Engage the inner thighs toward the midline to lift the pelvic floor and engage mula bandha. Maintain the soft sound of the breath through the contraction of the throat to gently apply jalandhara bandha.

5. Hold for as long as needed.

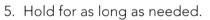

MUKTA HASTA SIRSASANA C
(MOOK-tah HAHS-tah sheer-SHAHS-anna)
mukta = liberated   hasta = hand   sirsa = head   asana = pose

TRIPOD HEADSTAND

First drishti: nasikagra—tip of the nose

1. From balasana (page 142), on an inhale, place your palms on the floor, shoulder-width apart with the fingers pointing forward. Place the top of the head between the hands. Extend the arms straight out to the side so they are in line with the top of the head. Turn the palms down and press through the hands to stabilize the shoulder girdle. Keep the arms engaged throughout this entire pose.

2. On an exhale, lift the knees off the ground and shift the weight to the head. Tip toe the feet in as close as possible, keeping both legs straight until the hips are over the shoulders.

3. On an inhale, lift both legs together or lift one leg and then the other, to come into a full inversion. The body is in a straight line, with weight primarily on the top of the head.

4. Draw the navel into the spine to engage uddiyana bandha, stabilize the core, and bring the breath into the rib cage. Engage the inner thighs toward the midline to lift the pelvic floor and engage mula bandha. Maintain the soft sound of the breath through the contraction of the throat to gently apply jalandhara bandha.

5. Hold for as long as needed.

BADDHA HASTA SIRSASANA A

(bahd-dah hahs-tah sheer-SHAHS-ahna)

baddha = bound   hasta = hand   sirsa = head   asana = pose

BOUND HAND HEADSTAND POSE

First drishti: nasikagra—tip of the nose

1. From adho mukha svanasana (page 56), drop the knees to the floor.

2. Drop the elbows to the floor, and place the top of the head on the floor. Interlace your fingers to cradle the back of the head in your open palms. Feel the top of the head pressing into the floor.

3. Lift the knees off the ground and shift the weight to the head. Tip toe the feet in as close as possible, keeping both legs straight until the hips are over the shoulders.

4. Lift both legs off the ground until the body is in a vertical line.

5. Draw the navel into the spine to engage uddiyana bandha, stabilize the core, and bring the breath into the rib cage. Engage the inner thighs toward the midline to lift the pelvic floor and engage mula bandha. Maintain the soft sound of the breath through the contraction of the throat to gently apply jalandhara bandha.

6. Hold for as long as needed.

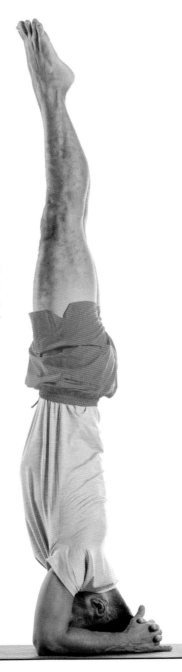

BADDHA HASTA SIRSASANA B

(bahd-dah hahs-tah sheer-SHAHS-ahna)

baddha = bound   hasta = hand   sirsa = head   asana = pose

BOUND HAND HEADSTAND POSE

First drishti: nasikagra—tip of the nose

1. From adho mukha svanasana (page 56), drop the knees to the floor.

2. Drop the elbows to the floor, and place the top of the head on the floor. Cross your arms in front of your forehead by first bringing the fingers of the right hand to hold the left biceps, placing the left forearm over the right forearm, then reaching the left fingers under the right biceps. Press the forearms and the top of the head firmly into the floor.

3. Lift the knees off the ground and shift the weight to the head. Tip toe the feet in as close as possible, keeping both legs straight until the hips are over the shoulders.

4. Lift both legs off the ground until the body is in a vertical line.

5. Draw the navel into the spine to engage uddiyana bandha, stabilize the core, and bring the breath into the rib cage. Engage the inner thighs toward the midline to lift the pelvic floor and engage mula bandha. Maintain the soft sound of the breath through the contraction of the throat to gently apply jalandhara bandha.

6. Hold for as long as needed.

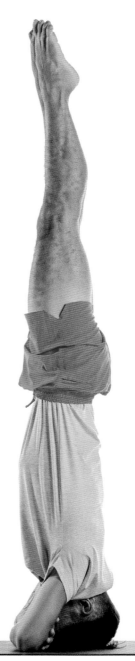

BADDHA HASTA SIRSASANA C

(bahd-dah hahs-tah sheer-SHAHS-ahna)

baddha = bound   hasta = hand   sirsa = head   asana = pose

BOUND HAND HEADSTAND POSE

First drishti: nasikagra—tip of the nose

1. From adho mukha svanasana (page 56), drop the knees to the floor.

2. Drop the elbows to the floor, bringing the forearms shoulder-width apart and parallel. Place the top of the head on the floor between the wrists. Press the forearms and the top of the head firmly into the floor.

3. Lift the knees off the ground and shift the weight to the head. Tip toe the feet in as close as possible, keeping both legs straight until the hips are over the shoulders.

4. Lift both legs off the ground until the body is in a vertical line.

5. Draw the navel into the spine to engage uddiyana bandha, stabilize the core, and bring the breath into the rib cage. Engage the inner thighs toward the midline to lift the pelvic floor and engage mula bandha. Maintain the soft sound of the breath through the contraction of the throat to gently apply jalandhara bandha.

6. Hold for as long as needed.

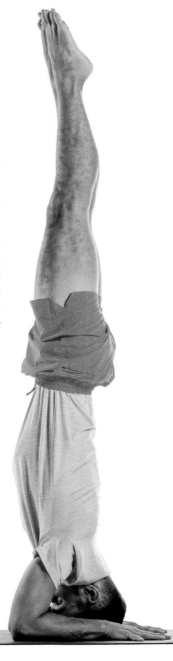

BADDHA HASTA SIRSASANA D

(bahd-dah hahs-tah sheer-SHAHS-ahna)

baddha = bound   hasta = hand   sirsa = head   asana = pose

BOUND HAND HEADSTAND POSE

First drishti: nasikagra—tip of the nose

1. From adho mukha svanasana (page 56), drop the knees to the floor.

2. Drop the elbows to the floor, bringing the forearms shoulder-width apart and parallel. Place the top of the head on the floor between the wrists, then bring the fingers to touch the back of the shoulders so that only the elbows are touching the ground. Press the elbows and the top of the head firmly into the floor.

3. Lift the knees off the ground and shift the weight to the head. Tip toe the feet in as close as possible, keeping both legs straight until the hips are over the shoulders.

4. Lift both legs off the ground until the body is in a vertical line.

5. Draw the navel into the spine to engage uddiyana bandha, stabilize the core, and bring the breath into the rib cage. Engage the inner thighs toward the midline to lift the pelvic floor and engage mula bandha. Maintain the soft sound of the breath through the contraction of the throat to gently apply jalandhara bandha.

6. Hold for as long as needed.

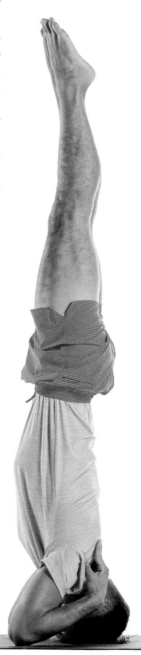

Inversion and Rest Postures (Finishing Series)

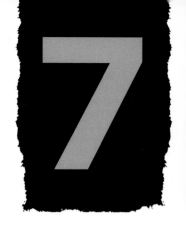

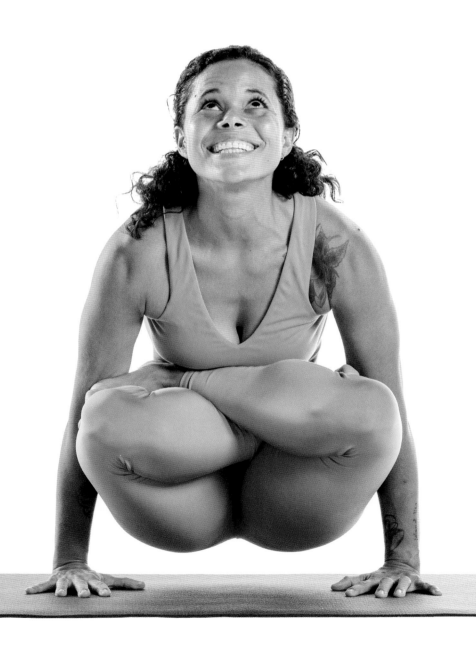

The postures featured in this chapter are performed as part of the final and finishing poses of classical ashtanga and the Rocket sequences (see chapters 8 and 9) and should be done with ease and as much relaxation as possible. The body has worked hard, and the finishing poses cool and calm the internal energy and prepare the body for the final rest—savasana.

The finishing series poses are held for longer counts of eight to ten slow, deep breaths. The inversions—sarvangasana and sirsasana—can be held for even longer, up to 20 breaths or more, if desired. Continue to apply the ujjayi breath here, bringing a more relaxed energy to the poses in order to tap into their cooling and restorative nature.

SALAMBA SARVANGASANA

(sah-LOM-bah sar-van-GAHS-anna)

sa = with   alamba = support
sarva = all   anga = limb   asana = pose

SHOULDER STAND

First drishti: nasikagra—tip of the nose

1. From adho mukha svanasana (page 56), come to a seated, straight-legged position.
2. Lie flat on the back.
3. Lift the legs and hips over the shoulders, and raise the legs up to the ceiling. Hands can support the lower back. Keep the toes, hips, and shoulders in one line straight up toward the ceiling.

Modifications

- If it is not possible to align the feet directly over the shoulders while keeping the spine straight, let the hips rest a little behind the shoulders and feet a little over the head.

- If you have a neck injury or you want to ease the pressure in the back and neck, practice viparita karani (legs up the wall pose). Lie on the floor with the hips as near the wall as possible, and straighten the legs up the wall. This can also be performed away from the wall by holding the legs perpendicular to the ground (see smaller figure).

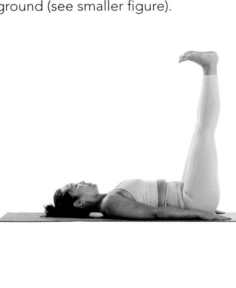

HALASANA

(hah-LAHS-anna)

hala = plow   asana = pose

PLOW POSE

First drishti: nasikagra—tip of the nose

1. From salamba sarvangasana (page 183), keep the legs straight and lower them above the head until the tops of the feet touch the ground. Point the toes.
2. Release the arms from the lower back, clasp the hands, and then lower the clasped hands to the ground.
3. Draw the navel into the spine to engage uddiyana bandha. Keep the spine as straight as possible. Continue to straighten the legs, and keep the feet pointed to engage the lower body.

Modifications

- For tight shoulders, use a strap to bind the hands.
- For a tight back or tight hamstrings, keep the hands on the lower back for support and let the legs hang. Wait for the feet to touch the floor before releasing the hands toward the ground.

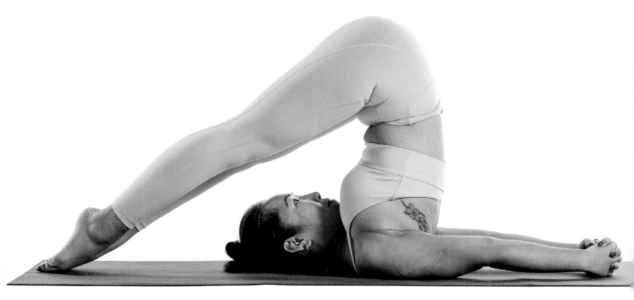

KARNAPIDASANA

(KAR-nah-peed-AHS-anna)

karna = ear   pida = pressure   asana = pose

EAR-PRESSURE POSE

DEAF MAN'S POSE

First drishti: nasikagra—tip of the nose

1. From halasana (page 184), bend the knees and separate the legs so the knees slide around the head.
2. Squeeze the knees onto the ears, and keep the hands clasped.
3. Keep breathing into the chest and as deeply as you can. Breathing against the compression of the posture causes the stretch to move from the inside toward the outside.

Modification

To ease the stretch in the back, bend the knees onto the top of the head. Leave the hands on the lower back for support.

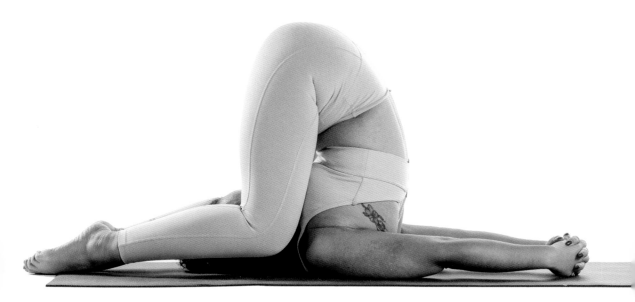

URDHVA PADMASANA

(OORD-vah pod-MAHS-anna)

urdhva = upward   padma = lotus   asana = pose

FLYING LOTUS POSE

First drishti: nasikagra—tip of the nose

1. From karnapidasana (page 185), bring the legs up to the ceiling as you support the lower back with the hands.
2. Take the legs into padmasana, with the right leg folding first.
3. Move the hands to the knees, and press the legs away from the chest until the arms are straight.

Modification

If the lotus position isn't possible, put the legs into an upside-down butterfly variation with the hands supporting the lower back (see smaller figure).

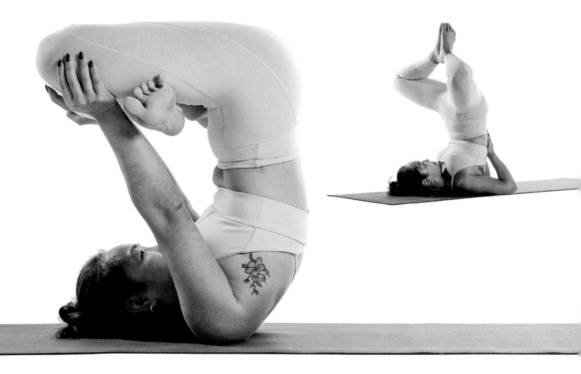

PINDASANA

(peen-DAHS-anna)

pinda = embryo   asana = pose

EMBRYO POSE

First drishti: nasikagra—tip of the nose

1. From urdhva padmasana (page 186), fold the legs at the hips, and bring the thighs into the chest.
2. Bind the hands around the thighs to pull in deeper.
3. Keep the balance on the back of the shoulders so the neck is relaxed and comfortable.

Modifications

- If binding around the lotus legs isn't possible, fold the full lotus into the chest by simply holding the knees. There is no need to bind.
- From butterfly variation, take the knees together and place them onto the forehead. Allow a little pressure to build on the third eye, the space between the eyebrows.

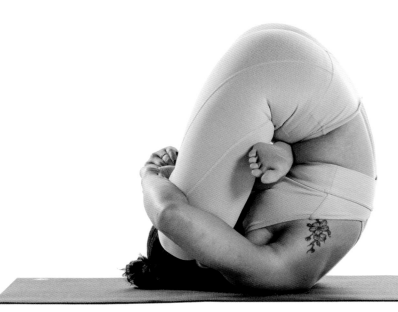

MATSYASANA

(mot-see-AHS-anna)

matsya = fish   asana = pose

FISH POSE

First drishti: nasikagra—tip of the nose

1. From pindasana (page 187), release the hands onto the floor toward the top of the mat.
2. Lower the body between the arms like two railroad tracks until the hips rest on the floor. Press the elbows strongly into the floor, and lift the chest to the sky.
3. Place the crown of the head on the floor to support and maintain the clean arch of the spine.
4. Grab the toes, and pull the lotus deeper.

Modifications

- If the lotus leg position is not possible, leave the legs in the butterfly variation. Feet stay together, and knees fall out to the side. Work on the arch of the spine from here.
- If the back extension is too intense, keep the legs in the butterfly variation, and the spine stays flat on the mat.

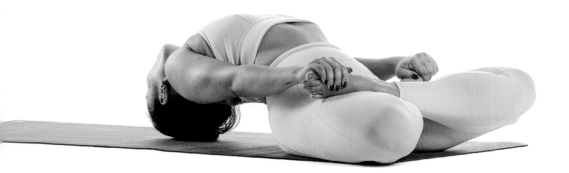

UTTANA PADASANA

(*oot-TAHN-a pod-AHS-anna*)

uttana = extended   pada = foot   asana = pose

EXTENDED-FOOT POSE

Second drishti: bhrumadhya—between the eyebrows (third eye)

1. From matsyasana (page 188), release the hands into prayer position, and release the legs from the lotus position.
2. Straighten the legs and arms, pressing the palms and toes together.

Modifications

- If the back can maintain the arch, release the legs onto the floor while keeping the arch of the spine.
- If the back cannot maintain the arch, flatten and relax the spine onto the floor. Keep the arms and legs reaching at a 45-degree angle.

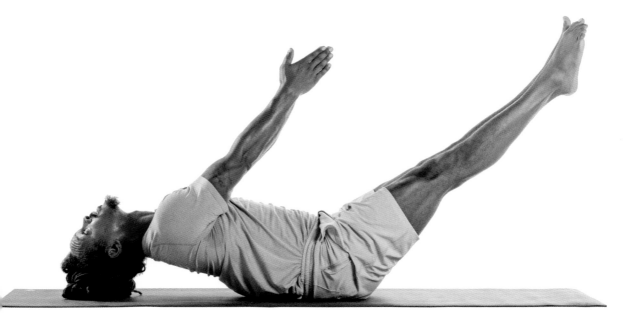

SIRSASANA

(shear-SHAHS-anna)

sirsa = head   asana = pose

HEADSTAND

First drishti: nasikagra—tip of the nose

1. From adho mukha svanasana (page 56), drop the knees to the floor.

2. Drop the elbows to the floor, and place the crown of the head on the floor. Clasp the back of the head with interlaced hands. Feel the crown of the head on the floor.

3. Straighten the legs, and walk the feet a little closer to the head so the hips rise over the shoulders.

4. Lift both legs off the ground until the body is in a vertical line.

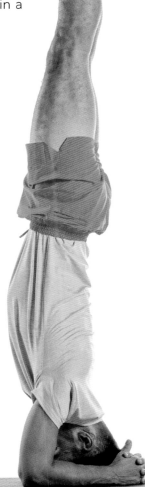

Modifications

These modifications address issues of balance as one works toward the full expression of the pose.

- Bend the knees and work on holding the headstand with the knees pulled into the chest (see figure a).
- Leave one foot or both feet on the floor and become comfortable with pressure in the head. Support the majority of the weight with the arms (see figures b and c).
- Use a wall to support the balance of the body, using the wall only to keep the body from falling over.

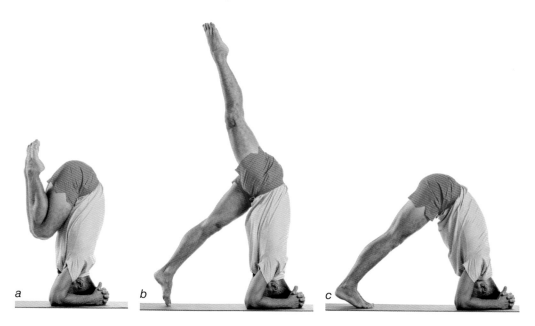

a   b   c

BADDHA PADMASANA/YOGA MUDRA

(BAH-dah pod-MAHS-anna) (YOH-gah MOO-drah)

baddha = bound   padma = lotus   asana = pose

yoga = union, yoke   mudra = seal, gesture

BOUND LOTUS POSE (SACRED SEAL)

First drishti: nasikagra—tip of the nose

1. From adho mukha svanasana (page 56), jump through to a seated position with the legs straight. Pull the legs into a full lotus with the right foot first. Work on taking the full bind with the right hand grabbing the right foot. The left hand grabs the left foot. This is baddha padmasana (see figure a).
2. On an inhale, look up to the sky and open the heart.
3. Exhale to fold forward placing the chin on the floor to enter yoga mudra (see figure b).

Modifications

- If the shoulders are tight, grab the elbows behind the back and fold forward.
- If the lotus leg position is not possible, cross the legs into a half lotus or easy seated posture. Hands can reach in front while you fold forward over the knees.

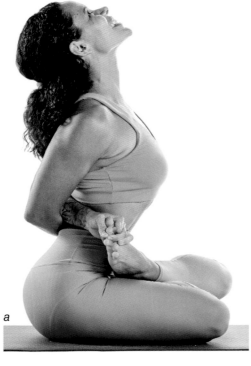

a

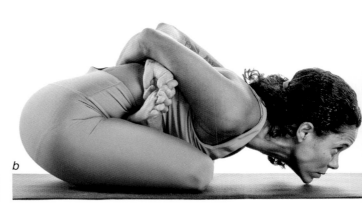

b

PADMASANA
(pod-MAHS-anna)
padma = lotus   asana = pose

FULL LOTUS

First drishti: nasikagra—tip of the nose

1. From baddha padmasana/yoga mudra (page 192), sit up while maintaining the bind and look up toward the sky.
2. Release the bind and place the back of the wrists on the top of the knees. Keep the arms straight as the shoulders draw down and the spine aligns over the hips.
3. Bring the fingers to yoga mudra by bringing the tip of the index finger to the tip of the thumb on both hands. Keep the other fingers straight.
4. Engage maha bandha to apply all three bandhas here. With each breath, focus on maintaining the integrity of the bandhas to move internal energy up the spine.

Modifications

- If the full lotus position is not possible, release the legs and take a comfortable seated posture.
- Use a block or pillow to raise the hips above the knees so the hips relax.

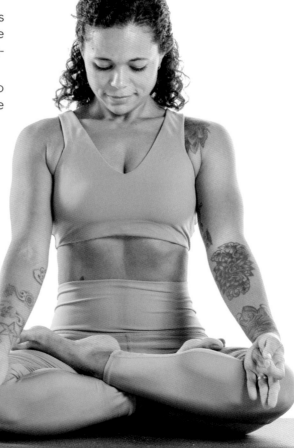

UTPLUTHIH
(*oot-PLOOT-tee-HEE*)
utplu = uprooting   thihi = stay or stand

SPRUNG-UP POSE

First drishti: nasikagra—tip of the nose

1. From padmasana (page 193), place the hands onto the floor outside and a little in front of the hips.
2. Press the hands into the ground, and lift the body off the floor. Pull the knees into the chest as the chin lifts toward the sky. Strongly engage the pelvic floor to help lift the body.

Modification

Release the full lotus posture. Work on lifting just the sitz bones off the floor and lifting the knees (see smaller figure). The feet can rest on the mat or help with the lift.

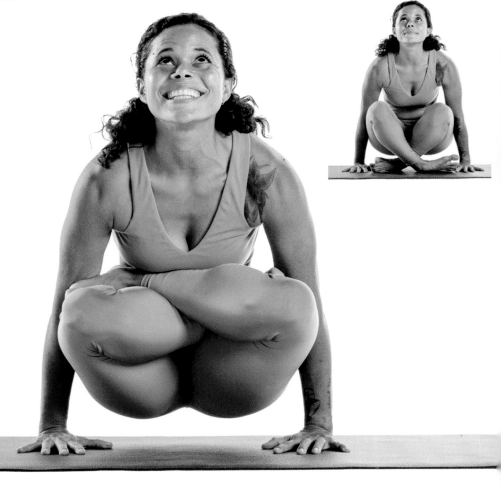

SAVASANA

(shuh-VAHS-anna)

sava = corpse   asana = pose

CORPSE POSE

Drishti: None, eyes are closed softly

1. Lie down and relax completely.
2. Allow the legs to splay open, and move the arms away from the body, palms facing upward.
3. Allow the breath to relax into its natural rhythm.
4. As the final resting pose, stay in this pose for five minutes or longer until your heart rate has returned to its resting rhythm.

Modifications

- For tightness in the lower back, place a pillow or bolster under the knees.
- For tightness in the neck and shoulders, place a small pillow under the neck.

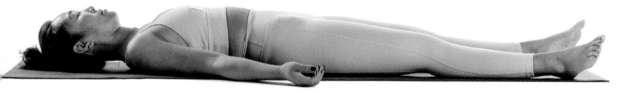

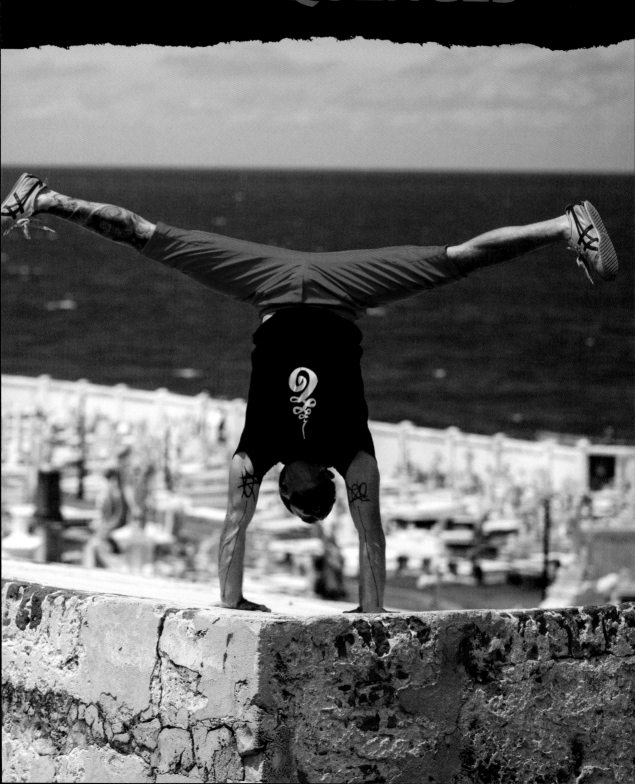

Classical
Ashtanga Series

8

Classical ashtanga is a dynamic and athletic form of hatha yoga composed of six series, each with a set sequence and a fixed order of postures. The practice is physically demanding and requires flexibility, strength, stamina, and a steady mind. Each of the six series begins the same way—warming up with surya namaskar A and B, followed by the standing series. After this, begin the series you are practicing for the day, whether it is the full primary, half intermediate, or full intermediate series. All practices end the same way, with the finishing series to cool the body.

Classical ashtanga is meant to be practiced six days a week, ideally at the same time each day. While some see the practice as rigid and demanding, the discipline built from this practice allows you to quickly see progress.

Sun Salutations

One of the oldest sequences of breath with movement, the surya namaskar (sun salutations) sequence accesses all of the muscles and joints in the body. This graceful mala of postures linked with breath can be both energetically grounding as well as invigorating, and it prepares the body for deeper practices by flushing the body with fresh blood flow, raising internal body temperatures, stimulating the nervous system, and opening the subtle body. These movements warm the physical body and begin to turn one's attention inward.

Sun salutations teach the details of breath and body coordination, a foundation that should not be skipped by students new to the practice nor by experienced practitioners. While the physical focus of surya namaskar A is to warm up the spine through movements of flexion and extension, surya namaskar B incorporates lunges that begin to move energy down through the hips and to the legs.

All classical ashtanga series begin with the sun salutations. Traditionally, five rounds of surya namaskar A are followed by three rounds of surya namaskar B, with each pose linked to a specific breath. For example, during surya namaskar A you exhale, samasthiti; inhale, urdhva hastasana; exhale, uttanasana; and so on.

Surya Namaskar A

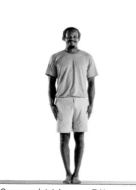

Samasthiti (page 51)

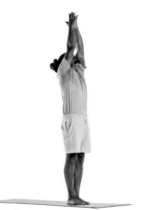

Urdhva Hastasana (page 52)

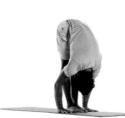

Uttanasana (page 70)

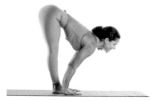

Ardha Uttanasana (page 72)

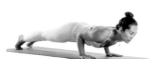

Chaturanga Dandasana (page 54)

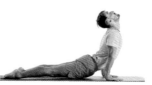

Urdhva Mukha Svanasana (page 55)

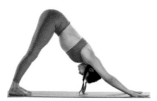

Adho Mukha Svanasana (page 56)

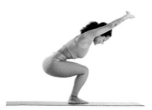

Ardha Utkatasana (page 58)

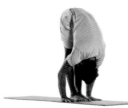

Uttanasana (page 70)

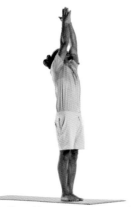

Urdhva Hastasana (page 52)

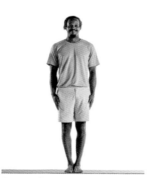

Samasthiti (page 51)

Surya Namaskar B

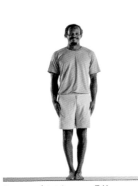

Samasthiti (page 51)

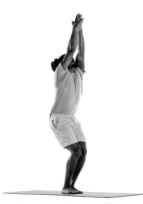

Utkatasana (page 57)

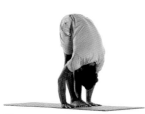

Uttanasana (page 70)

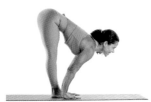

Ardha Uttanasana (page 72)

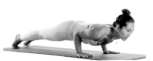

Chaturanga Dandasana
(page 54)

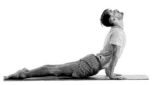

Urdhva Mukha Svanasana
(page 55)

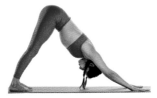

Adho Mukha Svanasana
(page 56)

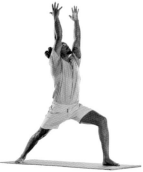

Virabhadrasana A (page 61)

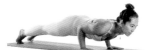

Chaturanga Dandasana
(page 54)

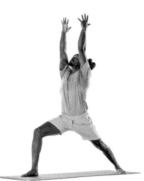

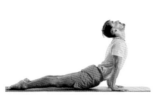

Urdhva Mukha Svanasana (page 55)

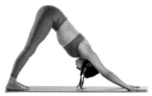

Adho Mukha Svanasana (page 56)

Virabhadrasana A (page 61)

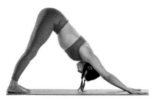

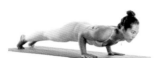

Chaturanga Dandasana (page 54)

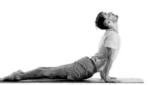

Urdhva Mukha Svanasana (page 55)

Adho Mukha Svanasana (page 56)

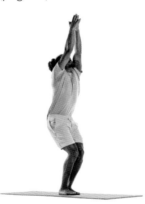

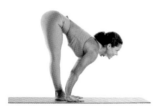

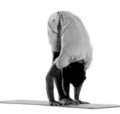

Ardha Uttanasana (page 72)   Uttanasana (page 70)

Utkatasana (page 57)

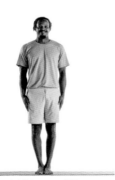

Samasthiti (page 51)

Standing Series

The standing series grounds the body by engaging the strength of the legs. The sequence of poses effectively warms up the legs and hips. Binding of the hands is optional but adds to the grounding nature of the sequence. All classical ashtanga series perform this standing sequence of postures after surya namaskar A and B. After you finish the final standing series pose, parsvottanasana, you go directly into the series you are practicing that day, whether it is full primary or intermediate.

Each pose is held for five long, ujjayi breaths. This provides enough time for the pose to unfold inside the body and for the body to receive the benefits of the pose.

Standing Series

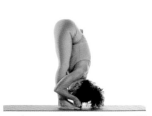
Padangusthasana (page 68)

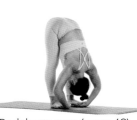
Padahastasana (page 69)

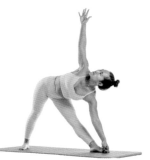
Utthita Trikonasana (page 63)

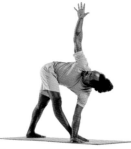
Parivrtta Trikonasana
(page 64)

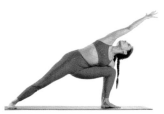
Utthita Parsvakonasana
(page 65)

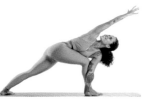
Parivrtta Parsvakonasana
(page 66)

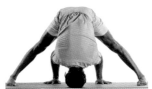
Prasarita Padottanasana A
(page 73)

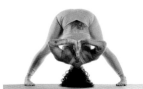
Prasarita Padottanasana B
(page 74)

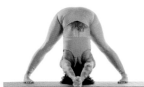
Prasarita Padottanasana C
(page 75)

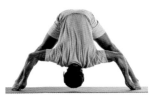
Prasarita Padottanasana D
(page 76)

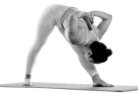
Parsvottanasana (page 82)

Primary Series

This is the first series of classical ashtanga vinyasa yoga as traditionally taught by Pattabhi Jois. It is often described as yoga therapy that creates discipline and consistency through the nature of the same rhythmic poses. Similar to a ritual, the traditional series follows an exact vinyasa count. The focus of this series is on the knees, hips, hamstrings, and spine and has more than 50 forward bends. The overall energetic effect of this series is to establish a sense of calmness and to relax and strengthen the muscles so the student can maintain a seated, still position for two hours or more.

This series was originally designed to maintain youthful energy through the mystical techniques of the ashtanga yoga lineage. Following the prescribed order of postures is required in a traditional setting; students are not allowed to practice a posture until they have completed the posture that comes before it. Ideally, this provides safety by requiring the body to open into one posture at a time. Each posture in the series prepares the student for the next one.

The half primary series stops the practice at navasana and moves directly into the finishing series as a complete practice. You can stop at half if you find the entire series too challenging, you are short on time, or you have not yet built the stamina to practice the entire series. The half primary series takes approximately 60 minutes to complete, while the full primary series takes 75 to 90 minutes.

Each pose is held for five long, ujjayi breaths. This provides enough time for the pose to unfold inside the body and for the body to receive the benefits of the pose.

Primary Series

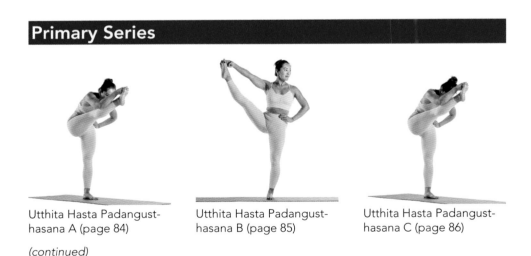

Utthita Hasta Padangust-
hasana A (page 84)

Utthita Hasta Padangust-
hasana B (page 85)

Utthita Hasta Padangust-
hasana C (page 86)

(continued)

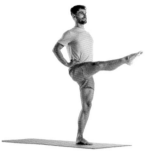

Utthita Hasta Padangust-
hasana D (page 87)

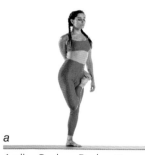

a

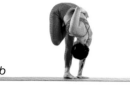

b

Ardha Padma Padmottanasana (page 88)

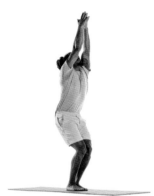

Utkatasana (page 57)

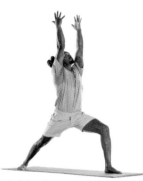

Virabhadrasana A (page 61)

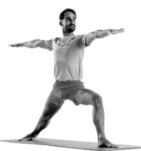

Virabhadrasana B (page 62)

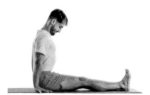

Dandasana (page 93)

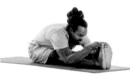

Paschimottanasana A
(page 94)

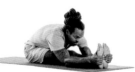

Paschimottanasana B
(page 95)

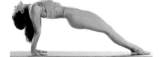

Purvottanasana (page 96)

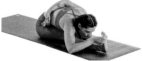

Ardha Baddha Padma
Paschimottanasana
(page 97)

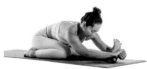

Trianga Mukhaikapada
Paschimottanasana
(page 99)

(continued)

Primary Series *(continued)*

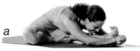
a

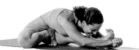
b

Janu Sirsasana A and B (page 100)

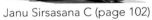
Janu Sirsasana C (page 102)

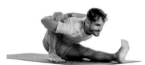
Marichyasana A (page 103)

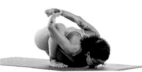
Marichyasana B (page 104)

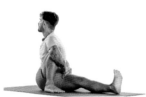
Marichyasana C (page 105)

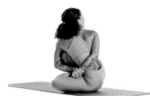
Marichyasana D (page 106)

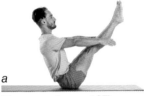
a
Navasana (page 107)

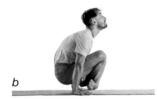
b

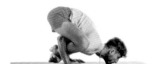
Bhujapidasana (page 109)

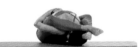
Supta Kurmasana (page 111)

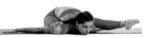
Kurmasana (page 110)

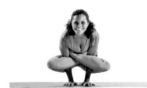
Kukkutasana (page 113)

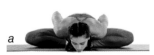
a
Baddha Konasana A and B (page 114)
b

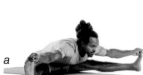
a

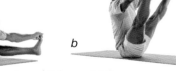
b

Upavistha Konasana A and B (page 116)

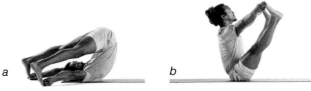

Supta Konasana A and B (page 118)

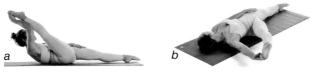

Supta Padangusthasana (page 120)

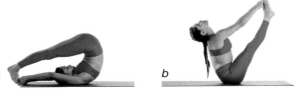

Ubhaya Padangusthasana (page 122)

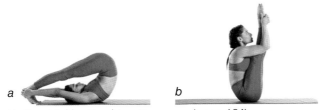

Urdhva Mukha Paschimottanasana (page 124)

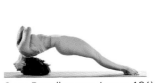 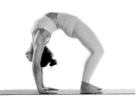

Setu Bandhasana (page 126)   Urdhva Dhanurasana
(page 128)

Intermediate Series

Known as nadi shodhana, meaning "nerve cleansing," this is the second of the classical ashtanga series. The intermediate series brings deep backbends, hip openers, and a series of inversions into the practice to open the energy channels, move prana, and challenge the body and the mind. The specific order of poses works directly on the nervous system. You will find that the intermediate series leaves a different energy than that of the primary series. The intermediate series can be challenging. Take the time to develop an awareness for each pose, keeping in mind that many modifications are available to help make the poses accessible.

The half intermediate series stops the practice after karandavasana. You can stop at half if you find the entire series too challenging, you are short on time, or you have not yet built the stamina to practice the entire series. The half intermediate series takes approximately 60 minutes, while the full intermediate series takes about 90 minutes.

Hold each pose for five long, ujjayi breaths. This provides enough time for the pose to unfold inside the body and for the body to receive the benefits of the pose.

Intermediate Series

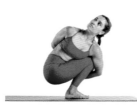

Pasasana (page 131)

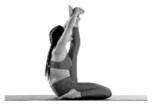

Krounchasana (page 135)

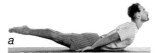

a   b

Shalabhasana A and B

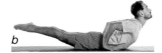

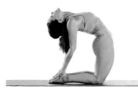

Bhekasana (page 140)

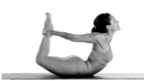

Dhanurasana (page 143)

(continued)

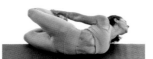

Parsva Dhanurasana
(page 144)

Ustrasana (page 146)

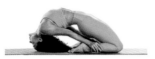

Laghu Vajrasana (page 147)

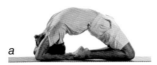

Kapotasana A and B (page 148)

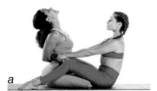

Supta Vajrasana (page 150)

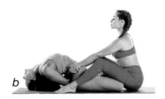

Bakasana A (page 60)

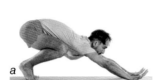

Bakasana B (page 152)

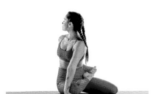

Bharadvajasana (page 155)

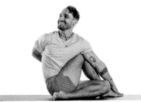

Ardha Matsyendrasana (page 156)

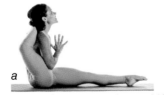

Eka Pada Sirsasana (page 163)

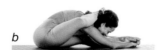

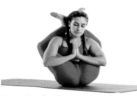

Dwi Pada Sirsasana (page 164)

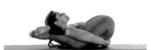

Yoga Nidrasana (page 165)

(continued)

Intermediate Series *(continued)*

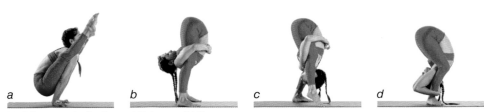

Titibhasana A, B, C, and D (page 166)

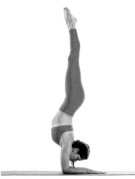

Pincha Mayurasana
(page 67)

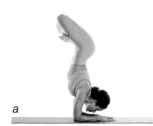

Karandavasana (page 168)

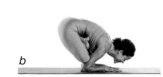

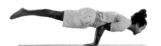

Mayurasana (page 169)

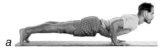

Nakrasana (page 170)

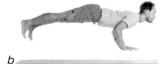

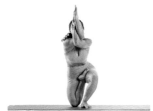

Vatayanasana (page 171)

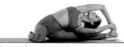

Parighasana (page 173)

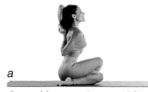

Gomukhasana (page 159)

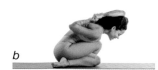

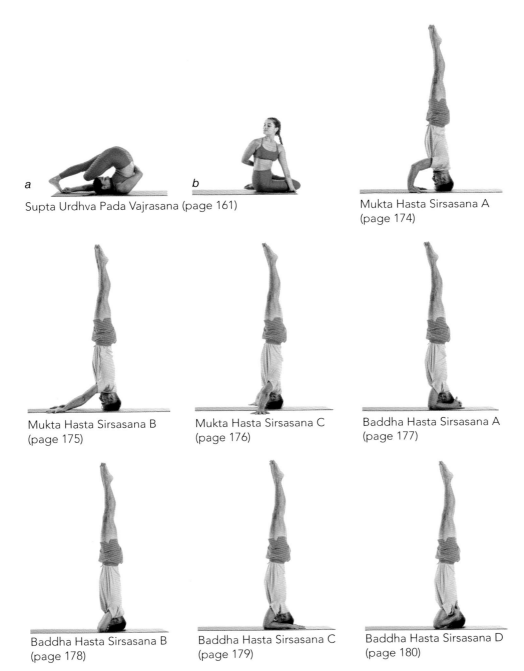

a
Supta Urdhva Pada Vajrasana (page 161)

b

Mukta Hasta Sirsasana A
(page 174)

Mukta Hasta Sirsasana B
(page 175)

Mukta Hasta Sirsasana C
(page 176)

Baddha Hasta Sirsasana A
(page 177)

Baddha Hasta Sirsasana B
(page 178)

Baddha Hasta Sirsasana C
(page 179)

Baddha Hasta Sirsasana D
(page 180)

Urdhva Dhanurasana (page 128)

Finishing Series

The finishing series is an important part of every classical ashtanga series. After surya namaskar A and B, the standing series, and the practice that day (half primary, full primary, half intermediate, or full intermediate), go directly into this finishing series to close your practice. It provides a set of inversions that reverse the blood flow in the body and allows the body to cool itself from within. This will refresh the body and bring harmony and balance back to the prana in the nadis, the energy channels inside the body. Allow time for the finishing series in every practice and hold poses for at least twice as long as the breath used during practice, extending the breath so it is slower and deeper. Finish with a mantra, personal prayer, or meditation on your highest intentions.

The finishing series poses are held for longer counts of 8 to 10 breaths. Continue to apply the ujjayi breath here, bringing a more relaxed energy to the poses in order to tap into their cooling and restorative nature.

Finishing Series

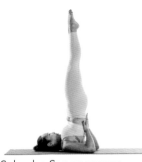

Salamba Sarvangasana
(page 183)

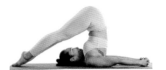

Halasana (page 184)

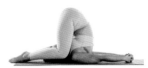

Karnapidasana (page 185)

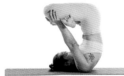

Urdhva Padmasana (page 186)

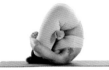

Pindasana (page 187)

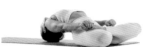

Matsyasana (page 188)

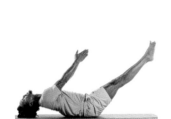

Uttana Padasana (page 189)

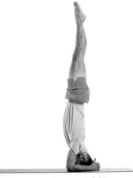

Sirsasana (page 190)

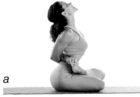

a

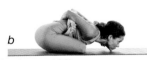

b

Baddha Padmasana/Yoga Mudra (page 192)

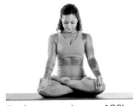

Padmasana (page 193)

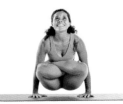

Utpluthih (page 194)

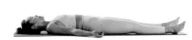

Savasana (page 195)

Original Rocket Yoga Series

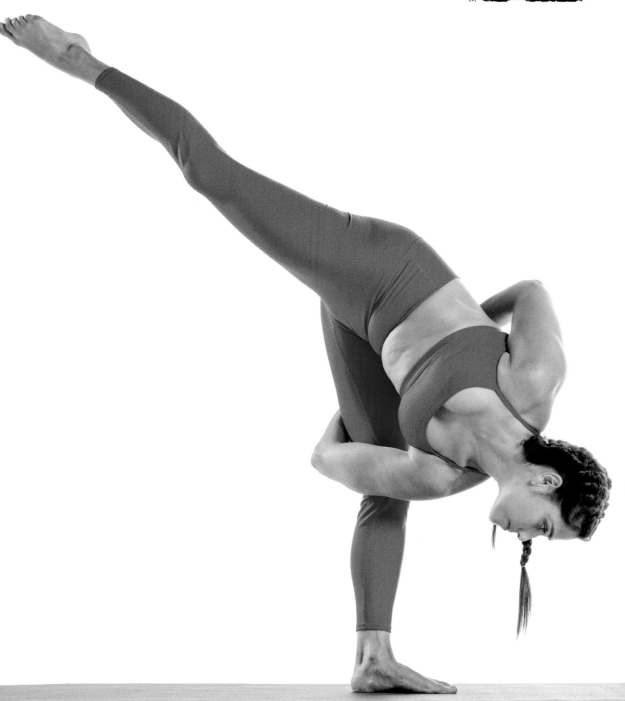

9

Rocket yoga is a clear distillation of the classical ashtanga series, from the format of the class to the breath count for each pose. It departs from the classical series in its reorganization of the standing asanas that offers more efficiency in tying together the standing sequence. This allows for more flow within the practice and adds a light and fluid energy. However, the poses themselves remain the same. In addition, Rocket yoga allows for more playfulness within the sequence, allowing you to insert nonclassical poses when the focus invites it.

In the seated series portion of the class, Rocket yoga omits many of the poses that can cause or exacerbate injury, such as the poses that require one or both legs to be in the lotus position. Additionally, many of the vinyasa transitions between poses are eliminated—again, to allow for more flow within the practice. The finishing series is much the same as in the classical ashtanga series; however, it demands less rigidity and offers options to students who may or may not want to close with the headstand and shoulder stand inversions. As you practice the classical ashtanga primary series, notice where Rocket yoga makes changes to this sequence and how that feels within your body.

Rocket I

Rocket I (also known as mixed levels) is a sequence modification of the standing series from classic ashtanga vinyasa yoga as well as a modified version of the seated series of the classic ashtanga primary series.

The Rocket standing series begins with utkatasana and brings the warrior postures to the front of the sequence in contrast to classic ashtanga, which ends the standing series with the warrior postures. Rocket I then guides you through a unique feature for leg strengthening, hip opening, and balancing by doing all poses on the right side first and then repeating on the left side. The standing poses are linked in a way that increases heat in the body as you move deeper into each pose. This technique speeds the process of strengthening the body while enhancing endurance and stamina by specifically stimulating the sympathetic nervous system while also maintaining proper bandha control to balance the parasympathetic nervous system. This produces a power state in which you are highly alert and extremely tranquil at the same time. The Rocket I seated series is the modified version of the classic ashtanga primary seated series. Inversions such as handstands and elbow stands are introduced as the subsequences and transitions begin to show themselves within the basic sequences.

Similar to the classic ashtanga series, each pose is held for five long ujjayi breaths. This provides enough time for the pose to unfold inside the body and for the body to receive the benefits of the pose. Move directly from one pose to the next, maintaining the inner heat that you've built within your body.

Rocket I

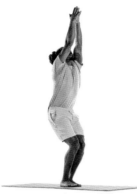
Utkatasana (page 57)

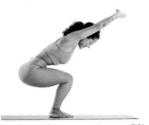
Ardha Utkatasana (page 58)

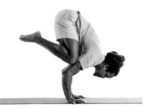
Kakasana (page 59)

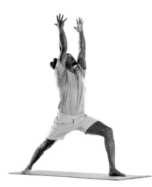
Virabhadrasana A (page 61)

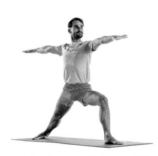
Virabhadrasana B (page 62)

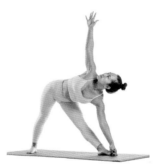
Utthita Trikonasana (page 63)

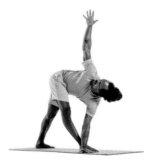
Parivrtta Trikonasana
(page 64)

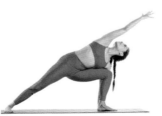
Utthita Parsvakonasana
(page 65)

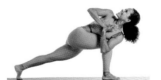
Parivrtta Parsvakonasana
(page 66)

(continued)

Rocket I *(continued)*

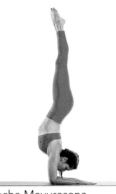

Pincha Mayurasana
(page 67)

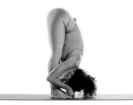

Padangusthasana (page 68)

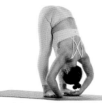

Padahastasana (page 69)

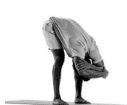

Uttanasana variation
(page 71)

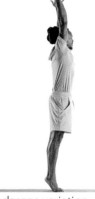

Tadasana variation
(page 53)

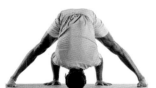

Prasarita Padottanasana A
(page 73)

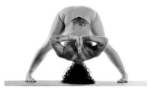

Prasarita Padottanasana B
(page 74)

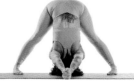

Prasarita Padottanasana C
(page 75)

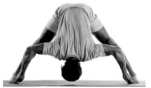

Prasarita Padottanasana D
(page 76)

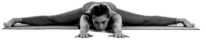

Samakonasana (page 77)

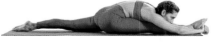

Hanumanasana (page 78)

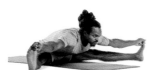

Upavistha Konasana A
(page 116)

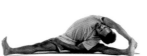

Upavistha Konasana varia-
tion (page 80)

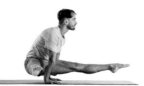

Mula Bandha Checkup
(page 81)

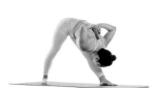

Parsvottanasana (page 82)

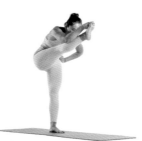

Utthita Hasta Padangust-
hasana A (page 84)

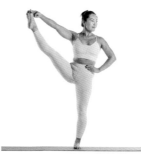

Utthita Hasta Padangust-
hasana B (page 85)

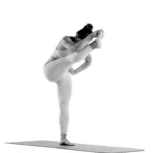

Utthita Hasta Padangust-
hasana C (page 86)

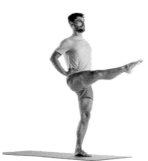

Utthita Hasta Padangust-
hasana D (page 87)

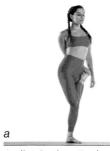

a

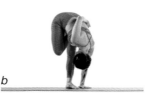

b

Ardha Padma Padmottanasana (page 88)

(continued)

Rocket I *(continued)*

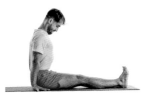
Dandasana (page 93)

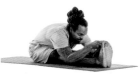
Paschimottanasana A (page 94)

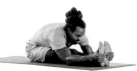
Paschimottanasana B (page 95)

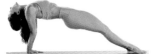
Purvottanasana (page 96)

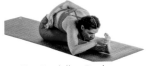
Ardha Baddha Padma Paschimottanasana (page 97)

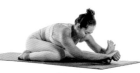
Trianga Mukhaikapada Paschimottanasana (page 99)

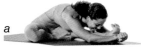
a

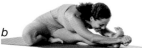
b

Janu Sirsasana A and B (page 100)

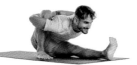
Marichyasana A (page 103)

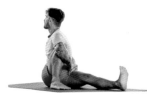
Marichyasana C (page 105)

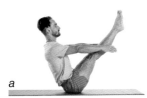
a

Navasana (page 107)

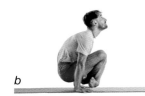
b

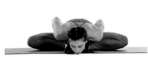
Baddha Konasana A (page 114)

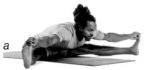
a

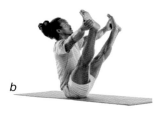
b

Upavistha Konasana A and B (page 116)

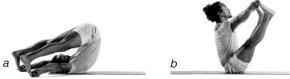
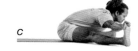

Supta Konasana A and B (page 118)

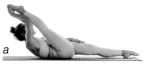
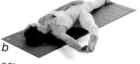

Supta Padangusthasana (page 120)

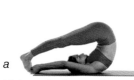
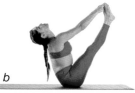

Ubhaya Padangusthasana (page 122)

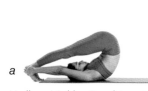
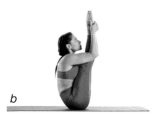

Urdhva Mukha Paschimottanasana (page 124)

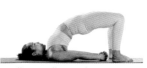
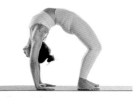

Ardha Urdhva Dhanurasana
(page 127)

Urdhva Dhanurasana
(page 128)

Rocket II

The Rocket II standing series uses the same classical ashtanga sequence modification as Rocket I, but omits the final standing postures, utthita hasta padangusthasana and ardha padma padmottanasana. The Rocket II standing series is designed to quickly prepare you to begin the seated series while still covering the fundamental standing postures.

The Rocket II seated series is a modification of the classical ashtanga intermediate series, starting from pasasana to the culminating headstands. You are introduced to various postures from the third, fourth, and fifth series of classical ashtanga. Through unique vinyasa transitions, you build body strength after all toxins and stiffness are released by practicing the primary series. It is a combination of nerve cleansing and awakening.

The tempo of Rocket II is a four-count inhalation and four-count exhalation. You can change this rhythm according to your level and knowledge. Slow the tempo if you're newer to the practice. A faster pace can be accomplished through shorter holds of the asanas. All transitions should be slow and controlled. Only the core postures of the series are held for five to eight counts. Most postures will be held for a three to five count.

While you are coordinating the breath and movements, the intention of this series is to become aware of the flow between postures—the transitions. Do not hold the postures for long periods, and modify them when breathing becomes difficult. This series is not designed to promote deep flexibility in postures, although that is an effect of the practice. Instead, the aim is to build strength within your body and encourage creativity within your practice.

The power of the poses and breath builds up the 11 main systems of the body, resulting in an optimal state of physical health and mental clarity. Respiratory, cardiovascular, muscular, skeletal, nervous, immune, digestive, excretory, endocrine, integumentary, and reproductive systems all play a role in the practice of ashtanga yoga. The practice awakens and charges the feeling body with the invisible energy of prana to bring the subtle experience of yoga to the practitioner.

Rocket II

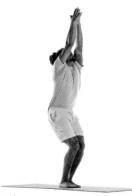

Utkatasana (page 57)

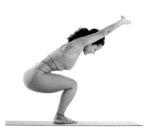

Ardha Utkatasana (page 58)

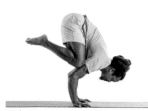

Kakasana (page 59)

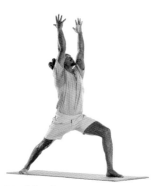

Virabhadrasana A
(page 61)

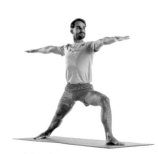

Virabhadrasana B (page 62)

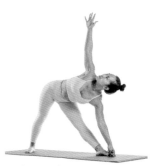

Utthita Trikonasana (page 63)

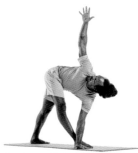

Parivrtta Trikonasana
(page 64)

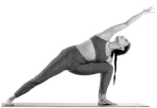

Utthita Parsvakonasana
(page 65)

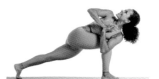

Parivrtta Parsvakonasana
(page 66)

(continued)

Rocket II *(continued)*

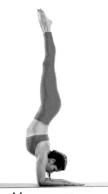

Pincha Mayurasana
(page 67)

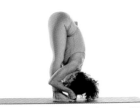

Padangusthasana (page 68)

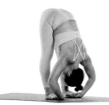

Padahastasana (page 69)

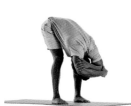

Uttanasana variation
(page 71)

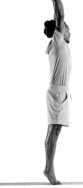

Tadasana variation
(page 53)

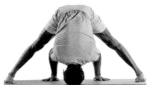

Prasarita Padottanasana A
(page 73)

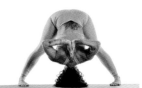

Prasarita Padottanasana B
(page 74)

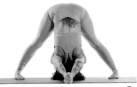

Prasarita Padottanasana C
(page 75)

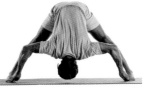

Prasarita Padottanasana D
(page76)

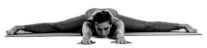

Samakonasana (page 77)

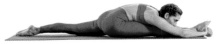

Hanumanasana (page 78)

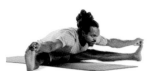

Upavistha Konasana A
(page 116)

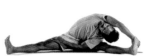

Upavistha Konasana varia-
tion (page 80)

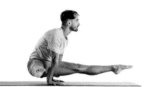

Mula Bandha Checkup
(page 81)

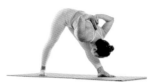

Parsvottanasana (page 82)

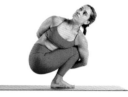

Pasasana (page 131)

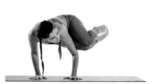

Parsva Bakasana (page 132)

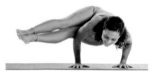

Dwi Pada Koundinyasana
(page 134)

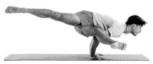

Parsva Koundinyasana
(page 133)

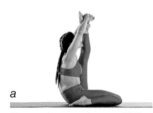

a   b

Krounchasana (page 135)

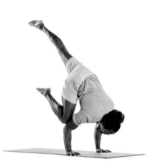

Eka Pada Bakasana
(page 136)

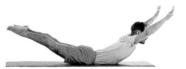

Astavakrasana (page 137)

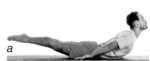

a   b

Shalabhasana A and B (page 138)

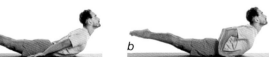

Shalabhasana variation (page 139)

(continued)

Rocket II *(continued)*

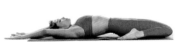

Supta Virasana (page 141)

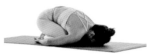

Balasana (page 142)

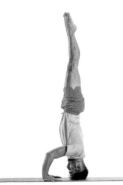

Mukta Hasta Sirsasana A
(page 174)

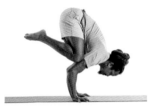

Kakasana (page 59)

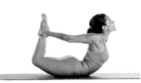

Dhanurasana (page 143)

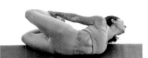

Parsva Dhanurasana
(page 144)

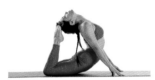

Raja Kapotasana (page 145)

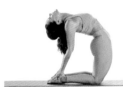

Ustrasana (page 146)

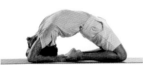

Kapotasana A (page 148)

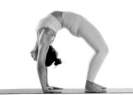

Urdhva Dhanurasana
(page 128)

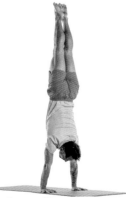

Adho Mukha Vrksasana
(page 154)

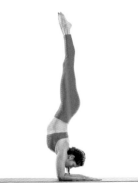

Pincha Mayurasana
(page 67)

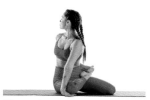

Bharadvajasana (page 155)

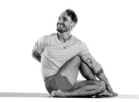

Ardha Matsyendrasana (page 156)

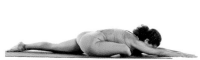

Adho Mukha Kapotasana (page 157)

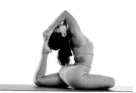

Eka Pada Raja Kapotasana (page 158)

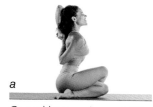

a

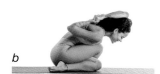

b

Gomukhasana (page 159)

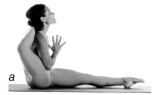

a

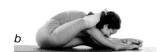

b

Eka Pada Sirsasana (page 163)

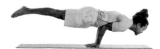

Mayurasana (page 169)

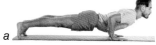

a

Nakrasana (page 170)

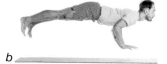

b

Rocket Arms and Legs

Rocket yoga classes can be structured to work on specific areas of the body. Within the sequence, add poses to strengthen the arms or poses that require more stamina from the legs. Use the instructions here as a guide to expanding the practice, or you can also use your creativity and add what feels best for your body at that moment.

Rocket Arms

The Rocket arms sequence strengthens the arms by focusing on transitions that strengthen the shoulder girdle and wrists and on stretches that increase the range of motion. This section lists common variations and transitions to add for a Rocket arms class.

Because these are variations of the poses, you may need more time to get into the pose or find that holding them for a full five breaths is challenging. Try to hold each pose for three to five long ujjayi breaths, remembering to breathe with intention during your transitions. It takes time for the body to receive the benefits of a pose, so be patient and breathe deeply.

You may feel a lot of sensation in your arms during this practice. Move directly from one pose to the next, maintaining the inner heat that you've built within your body.

Rocket Arms

Double push-up in sun salutations and vinyasas: After upward-facing dog, return to chaturanga, then push directly back into downward-facing dog.

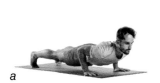
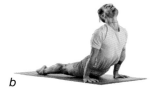
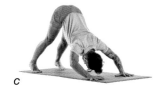

a   b   c

Plank core pumps in sun salutations: From downward-facing dog, inhale and lift one leg to the sky, maintaining the hip alignment squared to the ground. On an exhale, shift forward with shoulders to a high plank position as you simultaneously pull your knee to the forehead and thigh to chest. Separate your shoulder blades and tuck the tailbone. On an inhale, extend the leg back to the downward-facing dog position, stretching the leg to the sky. From here you can switch legs, or you can step the leg forward to warrior I.

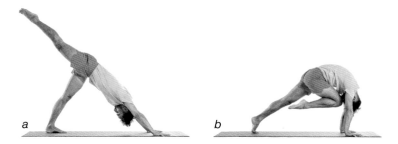

a   b

Handstand in sun salutations: After the half lift, press the hands into the mat and pike press into a handstand. Pike halfway down, then land in chaturanga.

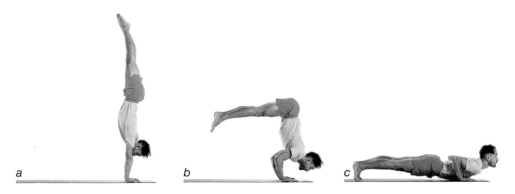

a   b   c

Arms bound behind the back in chair and half chair: Interlace the fingers behind the back, then stretch the arms straight and lift them off the body to stretch the front of the shoulders.

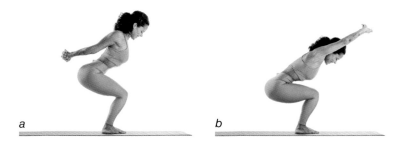

a   b

(continued)

Rocket Arms *(continued)*

Straight-arm crow and handstand crow: From crow pose, straighten the arms while keeping the knees tucked into the armpits. From here, press directly into a full handstand.

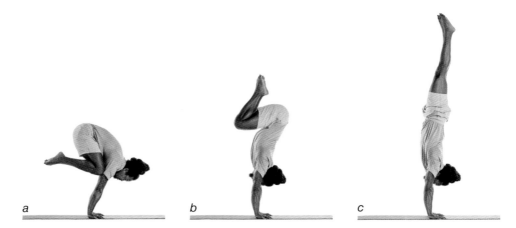

a   b   c

Arm bind in triangle: Bring the lower shoulder in front of the forward leg, then reach the same arm as the forward leg under and toward the lower back. Bring the top arm behind the back and bind the fingers or grab the opposite wrist. Straighten the arms as much as possible to stretch the front of the shoulders.

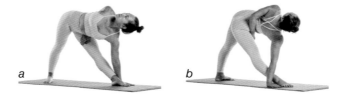

a   b

Sacrum check in revolving triangle: In revolving triangle pose, place the upper hand on the sacrum, checking that the hips are square and opening the shoulder to the ceiling before fully extending the arm.

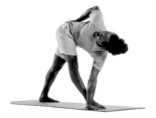

Bound extended-angle lunge: Bring the lower shoulder in front of the thigh of the forward leg, and reach the lower arm under the thigh and toward the lower back. Bring the top arm to the lower back, then grab the wrist with the other hand. Straighten the arms as much as possible to stretch the front of the shoulders.

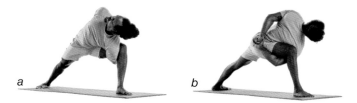

a   b

Revolving bound lunge: Bring the lower shoulder to the outside of the thigh of the forward leg, and reach the lower arm under the thigh and toward the lower back. Bring the top arm to the lower back, then grab the wrist with the other hand. Straighten the arms as much as possible to stretch the front of the shoulders.

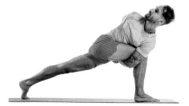

Forearm stand prayer and hollow back: From a steady forearm stand (pincha mayurasana), slowly begin to bring the chest through the upper arms to come into a hollow-back position.

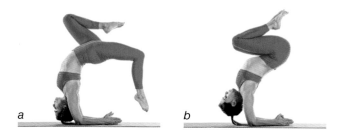

a   b

(continued)

Rocket Arms *(continued)*

Straddle press in wide-leg forward fold: From any variation of the wide-leg forward fold, bring the hands to the floor, shoulder-width apart. Press the hands into the ground, and press up into a handstand, moving through the straddle position.

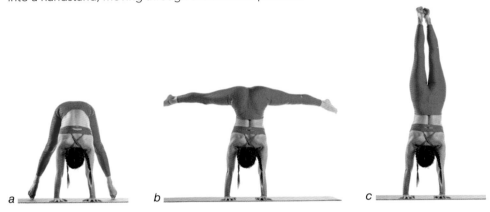

Side plank position out of full splits: With the right leg forward, place the left hand flat on the ground and even with the right knee. Grab the big toe of the right leg with the right hand, and lift the forward leg and the hips off the floor into a side plank position. This transition is reversed to seated splits.

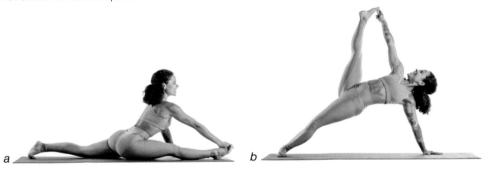

Full handstands in seated vinyasas: Instead of taking the most efficient transition in the seated vinyasas of the primary series, press up into a full handstand in the middle of each one.

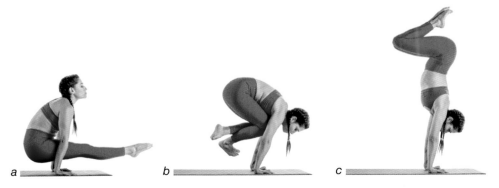

Rocket Legs

The Rocket legs sequence strengthens the legs and cultivates a grounding energy throughout the practice by adding variations to the standing series. This section lists common variations and transitions to add to a Rocket legs class.

Because these are variations of the poses, you may need more time to get into the pose or find that holding them for a full five breaths is challenging. Try to hold each pose for three to five long ujjayi breaths, remembering to breathe with intention during your transitions. It takes time for the body to receive the benefits of a pose, so be patient and breathe deeply.

This sequence is meant to be challenging for the legs, and you might feel a lot of sensation in your hips. That's OK. Move directly from one pose to the next, maintaining the inner heat that you've built within your body.

Rocket Legs

Chair pose with heels lifted: From any variation of chair pose, lift the heels off the ground as high as possible.

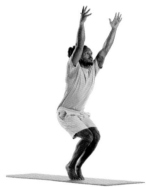

Crescent lunge after warrior I: After warrior I, pivot the back heel off the ground, and come to a crescent lunge.

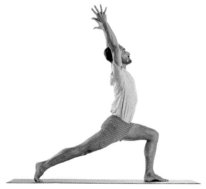

(continued)

Rocket Legs (continued)

Reverse warrior from warrior II: Keep the legs as they are, and reach the forward arm toward the ceiling and back. The back arm can reach down the back leg or can wrap behind the lower back, reaching to the opposite hip from behind.

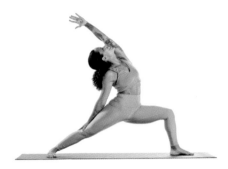

Standing split, half moon, and twisting half moon between triangles: From triangle pose, add this sequence, staying on the same standing leg before transitioning to the other side.

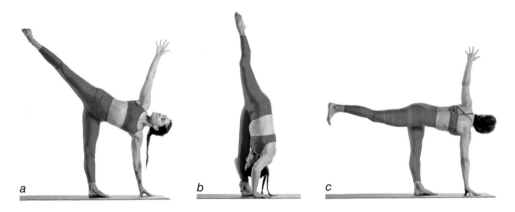

Bird of paradise and bound half moon after extended side angle: From extended side angle, bind around the forward leg. From here, come into either bird of paradise or bound half-moon pose.

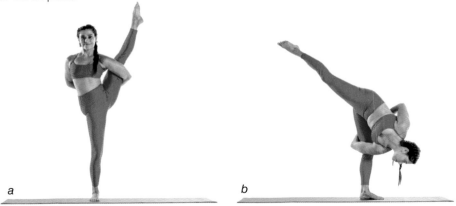

Revolving bird of paradise and half moon revolving bound after revolving extended side angle: From revolving extended side angle, bind around the forward leg. From here, come into either revolving bird of paradise or half-moon revolving bound pose.

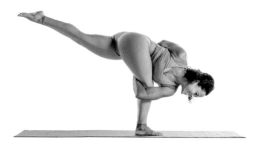

Bound side angle side plank transition to parsva koundinyasana: From a bound side angle, release the bind and place the bottom hand on the mat. Lift the forward foot and extend it straight forward, coming into a side plank variation. Keep the forward leg in this position as you bring the other hand to the ground, lifting the back leg off the floor to eventually come into parsva koundinyasana.

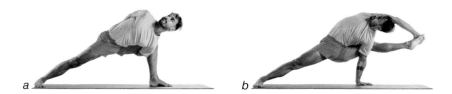

Full splits: Stay in this pose longer. You can add a bound twist under the legs or a backbend for variation.

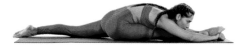

Pistol squats after utthita hasta padangusthasana D: Insert a pistol squat before moving into the half lotus forward fold.

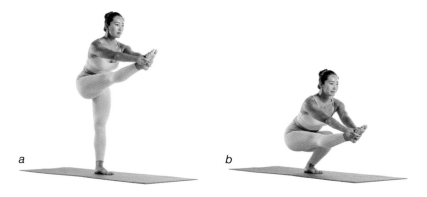

(continued)

Rocket Legs *(continued)*

Galavasana after half lotus forward fold: From half lotus forward fold, place both hands on the mat and bring the shin of the lotus leg to the upper arms. Lean forward and lift the back leg up to come into the arm balance, galavasana.

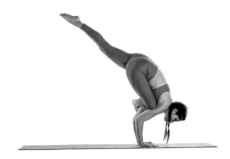

Rocket III

The week culminates in the Rocket III sequence, which combines all the poses you've practiced throughout the week. Also known as Happy Hour, Rocket III can be described as the combination of the Rocket I and Rocket II series, along with poses from the Rocket arms and Rocket legs series to form a practice that is fast paced and challenges your endurance. Because of this, you can also do it on days when your body is physically ready to push its limits.

The series begins the same as other Rocket classes, with sun salutations and the Rocket standing series, typically with the additional variations from Rocket arms and Rocket legs. This is followed by a modified primary seated series from Rocket I, and then you begin the Rocket II seated series after marichyasana C or after navasana. The finishing series follows as usual.

Rocket III offers both the hard and the soft forms of ashtanga vinyasa yoga in a clear and complete sequence that helps you to see the progression of the practice at the end of each week. Rocket III offers soothing forward folds and stimulating backbends in the same class. Bringing in many of the fun transitions from the ashtanga series, this exhaustive practice is a favorite for many students because it includes something for everyone, from backbending to inversions, working every part of the body. It is best practiced before a rest day to allow time for the body to recuperate from the long practice.

Rocket III

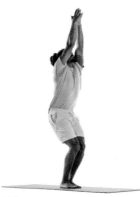

Utkatasana (page 57)

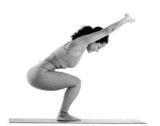

Ardha Utkatasana (page 58)

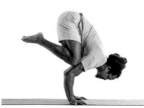

Kakasana (page 59)

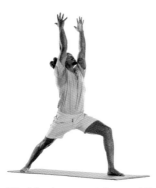

Virabhadrasana A (page 61)

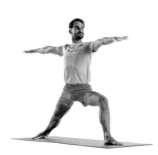

Virabhadrasana B (page 62)

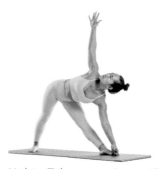

Utthita Trikonasana (page 63)

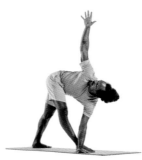

Parivrtta Trikonasana
(page 64)

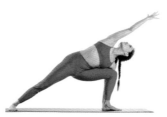

Utthita Parsvakonasana
(page 65)

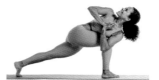

Parivrtta Parsvakonasana
(page 66)

(continued)

Rocket III *(continued)*

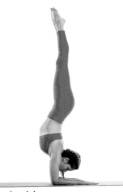

Pincha Mayurasana (page 67)

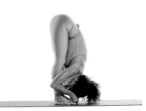

Padangusthasana (page 68)

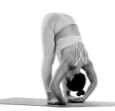

Padahastasana (page 69)

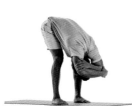

Uttanasana variation (page 71)

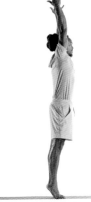

Tadasana variation (page 53)

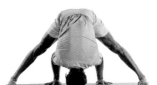

Prasarita Padottanasana A (page 73)

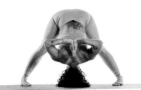

Prasarita Padottanasana B (page 74)

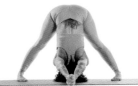

Prasarita Padottanasana C (page 75)

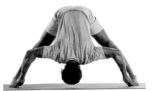

Prasarita Padottanasana D (page 76)

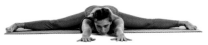

Samakonasana (page 77)

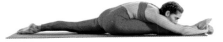

Hanumanasana (page 78)

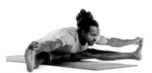

Upavistha Konasana A
(page 116)

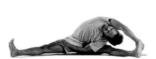

Upavistha Konasana varia-
tion (page 80)

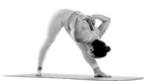

Parsvottanasana (page 82)

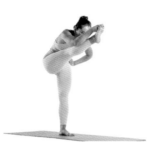

Utthita Hasta Padangust-
hasana A (page 84)

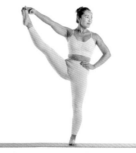

Utthita Hasta Padangust-
hasana B (page 85)

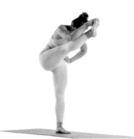

Utthita Hasta Padangust-
hasana C (page 86)

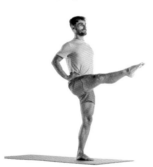

Utthita Hasta Padangust-
hasana D (page 87)

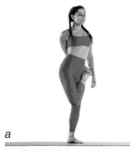

a

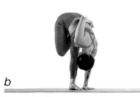

b

Ardha Padma Padmottanasana (page 88)

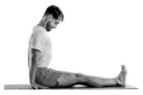

Dandasana (page 93)

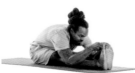

Paschimottanasana A
(page 94)

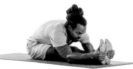

Paschimottanasana B
(page 95)

(continued)

Rocket III *(continued)*

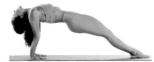

Purvottanasana (page 96)

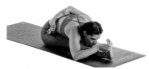

Ardha Baddha Padma
Paschimottanasana
(page 97)

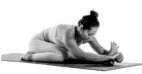

Trianga Mukhaikapada
Paschimottanasana
(page 99)

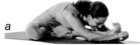

Janu Sirsasana A and B (page 100)

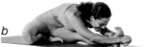

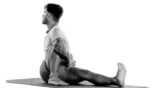

Marichyasana A (page 103)

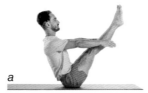

Marichyasana C (page 105)

Navasana (page 107)

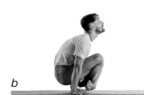

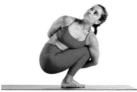

Pasasana (page 131)

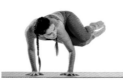

Parsva Bakasana
(page 132)

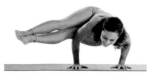

Dwi Pada Koundinyasana
(page 134)

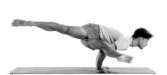

Parsva Koundinyasana
(page 133)

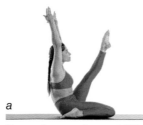

Krounchasana (page 135)

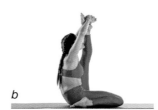

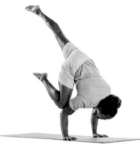

Eka Pada Bakasana
(page 136)

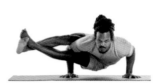

Astavakrasana (page 137)

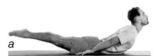

Shalabhasana A and B (page 138)

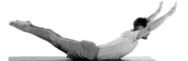

Shalabhasana variation
(page 139)

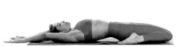

Supta Virasana (page 141)

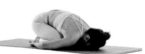

Balasana (page 142)

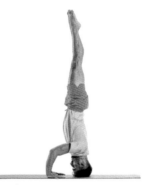

Mukta Hasta Sirsasana A
(page 174)

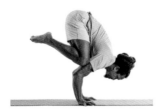

Kakasana (page 59)

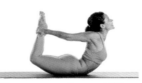

Dhanurasana (page 143)

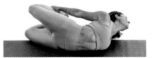

Parsva Dhanurasana
(page 144)

(continued)

Rocket III *(continued)*

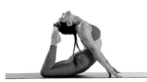
Raja Kapotasana (page 145)

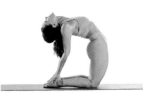
Ustrasana (page 146)

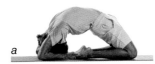
Kapotasana A and B (page 148)

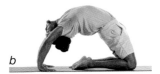

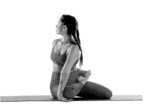
Urdhva Dhanurasana
(page 128)

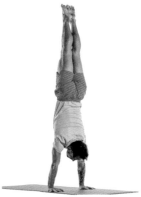
Adho Mukha Vrksasana
(page 154)

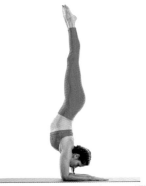
Pincha Mayurasana (page 67)

Bharadvajasana (page 155)

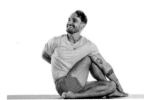
Ardha Matsyendrasana
(page 156)

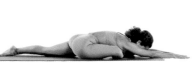
Adho Mukha Kapotasana (page 157)

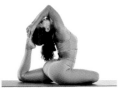
Eka Pada Raja
Kapotasana (page 158)

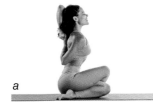
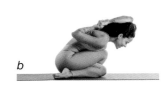
Gomukhasana (page 159)

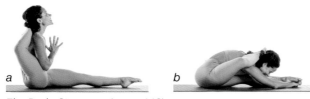

Eka Pada Sirsasana (page 163)

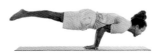

Mayurasana (page 169)

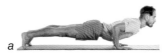

Nakrasana (page 170)

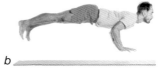

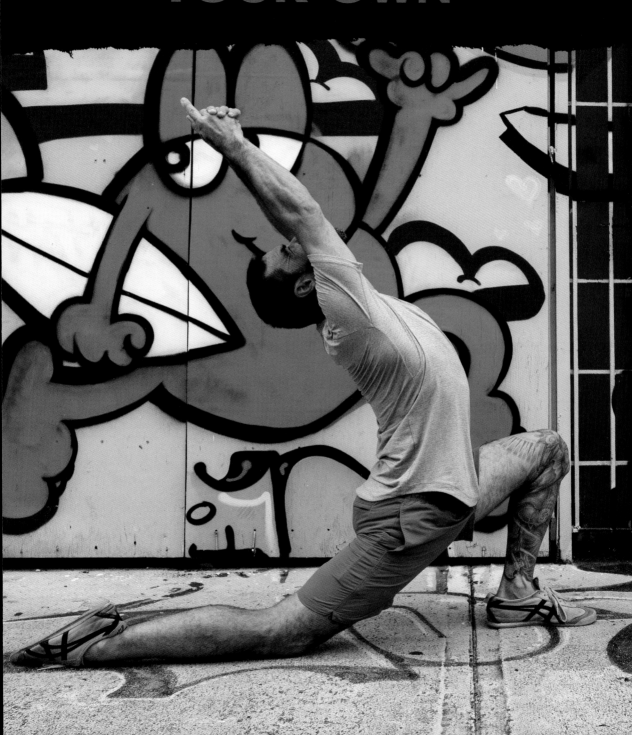

PART IV
MAKE THE PRACTICE YOUR OWN

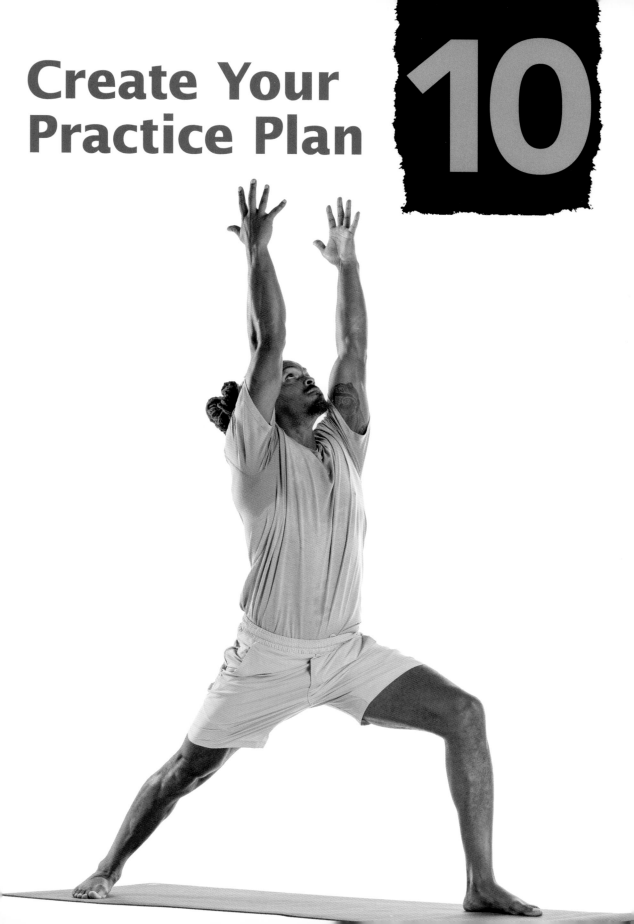

Create Your Practice Plan

10

The progressive ashtanga vinyasa method is meant to be practiced six days a week using a combination of the five series presented in chapters 8 and 9 (full primary, intermediate, Rocket I, Rocket II, and Rocket III), according to how you feel or how you would like to feel each day. It is up to you to decide how you would like to practice each day; however, you are encouraged to understand the benefit of not overexerting the body. The progressive ashtanga method is the practice of using both classical ashtanga and Rocket yoga to create a balanced weekly schedule that provides structure as well as freedom, discipline, and creativity.

Scheduling Your Practice

The five series—full primary, intermediate, Rocket I, Rocket II, and Rocket III—are evenly distributed throughout the week to encourage a soft and direct process of opening the body. Saturday is considered the day of rest, but you can choose any day to take rest.

All of the series treat the body as a whole, but each one has a specific focus on key areas of the body. These key areas are worked individually throughout the week in order to avoid overworking and provide a day of rest to let the muscles and joints recover, rebuild, and strengthen. You may repeat the Rocket I or Rocket II series during the week by using variations to the base sequence such as Rocket arms or Rocket legs. Full primary and a modified version of primary may be used interchangeably depending on individual ability level.

Committing to Your Practice

While practice is recommended six days a week, most practitioners need to work up to this level. If you do not already have a physical daily practice, it is not recommended that you go directly into practicing six days a week.

Start by committing to three days a week. Three days is enough to feel the benefits of the practice and build the stamina needed to add to your practice. By practicing every couple of days, your body will also retain the benefits from your previous practice. It is difficult to see progress in your own practice if you practice fewer than three days a week. If you can practice only three times a week or less, practice the classic ashtanga primary series (either modified or half primary) or practice Rocket 1. Try to practice at the same time each day. Creating a ritual will help to ingrain the practice into your daily life. Once you are comfortable practicing three times a week and you begin to see improvements with the flow and sequence of the practice, add a day. You will know if adding another practice is right when you have the energy to do another practice, you are not overly sore from the previous practice, and you mentally feel ready to do more. Work your way to six days a week, remembering that there is always one day off each week, and moon days or ladies holidays can be observed (moon days and ladies holidays are discussed in chapter 11).

Sample Practice Schedule When Practicing Three Days a Week

Sunday	Monday	Tuesday	Wednesday	Thursday	Friday	Saturday
Rest	Classic ashtanga or Rocket I	Rest	Classic ashtanga or Rocket II	Rest	Classic ashtanga or Rocket III	Rest

Sample Practice Schedule When Practicing Six Days a Week

Sunday	Monday	Tuesday	Wednesday	Thursday	Friday	Saturday
Classic ashtanga or Rocket I	Classic ashtanga or Rocket I	Classic ashtanga or Rocket II	Classic ashtanga or Rocket II	Classic ashtanga or Rocket III	Classic ashtanga or Rocket III	Rest

Your Practice Plan

Whether for yourself or for your students, outlining a weekly practice plan can help ensure that all parts of the body are focused on. Start with how many days you plan to practice. Write down which series you plan to practice each day.

Sunday	Monday	Tuesday	Wednesday	Thursday	Friday	Saturday

Fulfilling Your Minimum Daily Requirements

Although it is a physically and mentally demanding practice, ashtanga yoga is meant to be practiced daily. However, there will be days that you simply do not feel physically or mentally up to the challenge of a full practice. You may feel too sore from a previous day's events, or you may be emotionally drained. Your energy level might feel unusually low, or you may not feel mentally focused enough to stay on your mat to practice. It is important to honor how you feel—both physically and mentally, both on the mat and in your daily life. Staying authentic and honest about your needs is consistent with the practice of yoga. On days when your body does not feel its strongest or when you are recovering from an injury, set minimum daily requirements (MDR) as a simple way to stay connected to your practice and to your inner self. Here are the MDR:

- Surya namaskar A (do three to five rounds; page 201)
- Surya namaskar B (do three to five rounds; page 202)
- Paschimottanasana (page 94)
- Ardha urdhva dhanurasana (page 127)
- Savasana (page 195)
- Seated meditation (use the final three poses of the finishing series, which are considered the "seated meditation" portion of the classical ashtanga series; page 193)

When the body is not able to perform the MDR, it is recommended to practice the four purifications, a routine consisting of pranayama and kriya practices that can be practiced daily. These can be found in chapter 2.

Mind–Body Journaling

All philosophies that have existed across time began with a question. The only people who can answer these questions are the individuals who live within the questions. To notice change and progress inside your practice, it is crucial to write down the experiences and observations that arise.

Write down all of the questions that come to mind before or during practice. There is no need to answer the questions immediately, because that is what the practice is for! As you move through your physical practice, tapping into your intuition, the answers to some of your questions may become clearer to you. This is part of an exercise called "living in the question."

Keep a small journal you can use while you are in teacher training, anytime you change or add to your practice, or anytime you have questions. Write in this journal for 15 to 30 minutes after each practice while the experience and what you are feeling are still fresh in the body and mind. This is the best time to write down and contemplate the finer details of the practice, to find clarity in your questions, and to understand the answers that may appear.

In the space below, start by writing a few questions you may have regarding Rocket yoga or the progressive ashtanga vinyasa method. After your next practice, come back and reflect on your questions.

_____

_____

_____

_____

_____

Customize
Your Practice

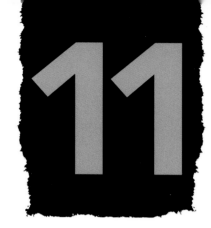

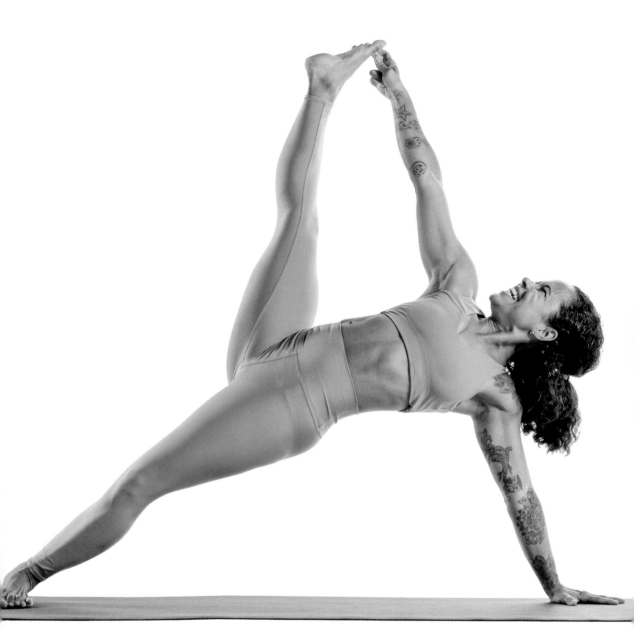

Everyone has unique strengths and their own challenges to overcome. There are many ways to tailor your practice to meet you where you are in your physical abilities and many ways your practice can accommodate you through different phases of life. Whether you need modifications to account for limited mobility or drills to build more strength, know that your practice can be amended to suit you.

Softening the Practice

Rocket yoga is designed to make the classical ashtanga vinyasa methods accessible to the masses. This is done by taking a softer approach that does not require binding or deep stretching of the joints and muscles. Rocket yoga brings freedom of movement and more space to allow you to take what serves you at the moment. Allow yourself to let go of the binds and rigidity of the practice. Turn your focus to the depth of the breath rather than the depth of the pose. Props and straps can be used when needed to complete the feeling of binds without pushing the body beyond its limit.

Here are a few suggestions for common modifications to soften the practice.

Modifications for Tight Hamstrings

- Bend your knees while in standing forward folds to lighten the stretch on the hamstrings, or place the hands at your feet or shins instead of the floor.
- Use a block to raise the floor when you need to push down into the ground. Enabling your hands to touch something, whether it's your shins or a block, helps you feel a sense of grounding.
- In seated poses, bend the knee of the leg that is being stretched, lengthening the lower back before stretching forward. If there is still discomfort, raise your seat by sitting on a block or bolster.
- Use a strap or towel to be able to reach the foot in seated poses.

Modifications for Tight Shoulders

- If the shoulders are tight or lack overhead external rotation, keep the hands shoulder-width apart or wider when reaching overhead instead of touching the palms together. Use the extra space to draw the shoulder blades down the back, allowing the arms to be supported by the back body.
- In poses where the arms are extended to the sides (example: warrior II), turn the palms upward to relieve tightness in the shoulders by opening across the chest and allowing the arms to be supported by the back body.
- Use a strap or hand towel to help with binds that require shoulder flexibility. When using a strap for binds, try to hold it in the top hand, allowing gravity to guide it to the lower hand. In seated poses that

use a bind, hold the towel in the hand of the arm that is more free, and swing it over to the other hand. Open the chest in binds that are behind the back, even when using a strap or towel to modify.

Modifications for Wrist Pain

It's common in the beginning stages to experience wrist discomfort, and this can hinder the process for many students looking to master the vinyasa technique. If you begin to feel discomfort, then take a look at modifications that will avoid making the problem worse. Also, being knowledgeable of preventative measures for when you begin to move into the classical transitions such as chaturanga (push-up) and jump throughs will help to mitigate issues as you practice.

- If there is enough discomfort to cause pain when bearing weight on the wrist, use small push-up bars to neutralize the wrists.
- Use the fists or fingertips rather than a flat palm; however, this should be used cautiously. Although this modification relieves the wrist compression, it provides little stability and can leave the wrist vulnerable to further injury.
- Remove push-ups or inversions from your practice for a few days or longer in order to rest. Weight-bearing wrist positions are used in only a few postures within the series.
- If you have a predisposition to weaker wrists or are working with a previous wrist injury, you may find support for the wrists to be essential for a vinyasa practice that works deeply on the floor and with inversions. A wrist brace or wrap that alleviates pressure is recommended.
- Strengthen your hands and wrists through small exercises and stretches specifically designed to prepare you for your practice. Learn to slowly increase the stabilization and support around the wrist area.

Modifications for Balance

- Keep the feet hip-width apart for standing asana instead of together for better balance. In poses such as warrior I, the feet can also be aligned with the hips (standing on train tracks) instead of in one line (standing on a tightrope).
- In one-leg standing poses, a slight bend in the knee of the standing leg can help with balance by engaging the leg muscles and bringing the center of gravity lower.

Modifications for Vinyasa

- In the chaturanga movement, bring the knees to the floor before bending the elbows. You can also come all the way down to the belly during the push-up position.
- For the backbend, modify by using low cobra instead of a full upward-facing dog.

- You can move through child's pose to downward-facing dog or move through a tabletop position and step the feet back one at a time to get into downward-facing dog.
- For the seated vinyasas, remove the seated vinyasa technique and replace it with a simple lift by pressing both hands into the ground and lifting the hips and feet off the ground. You can alternatively do navasana (boat pose) during this transition to engage the core and bandhas.

Adding Challenging Variations or Transitions

While each transition is carefully prescribed within the classical ashtanga practice, Rocket yoga allows you to play with how you move from one asana to the next. For example, jumping or pressing up into a handstand during vinyasas is allowed to add creativity and difficulty within the practice. Or adding arm balances where they come naturally can offer a way to experiment with your practice and push your edge.

> "The sky is not the limit when you're flying a Rocket ship!"
>
> —Larry Schultz

Creativity can be applied to the fundamental postures themselves, such as taking a bind inside the extended side angle or changing the classical variation of the posture to bring more emphasis to different areas of the body. New postures can be added to the sequence to build on the fundamental asanas. For example, a common addition to the standing series is the posture ardha chandrasana or half-moon pose. This posture can be placed between the triangle postures and used as an additional challenge to build stronger and more stable legs.

Here are a few examples of transitions you can integrate within the practice. Even if you cannot quite do the full transition, remember that the important thing is to try your best and have fun while you move.

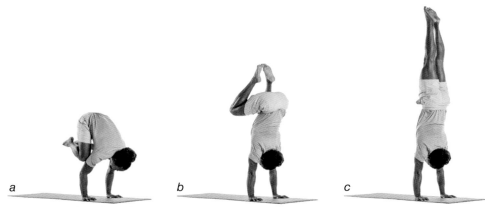

a   b   c

Bakasana to handstand

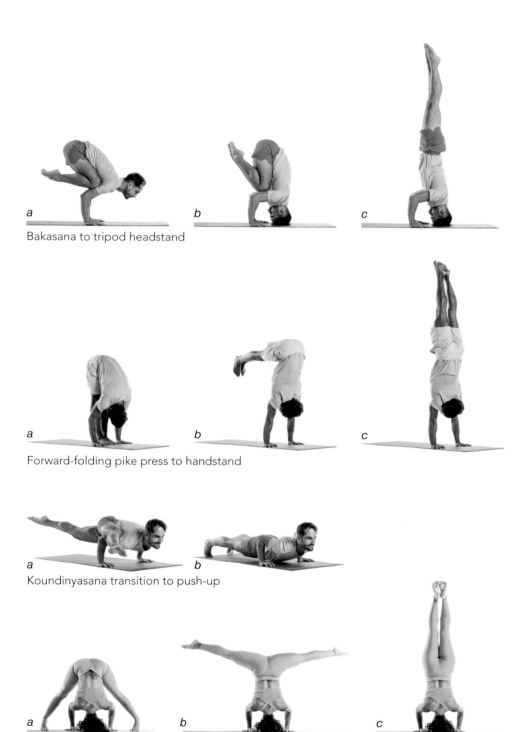

a   b   c

Bakasana to tripod headstand

a   b   c

Forward-folding pike press to handstand

a   b

Koundinyasana transition to push-up

a   b   c

Straddle press to headstand

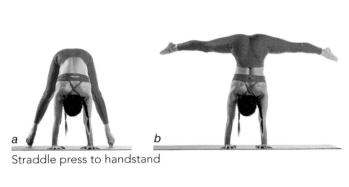
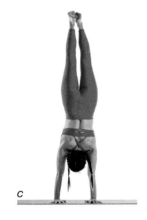

Straddle press to handstand

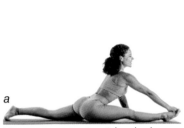
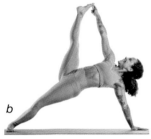
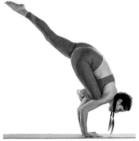

Hanumanasana to side plank

Standing half lotus to galavasana

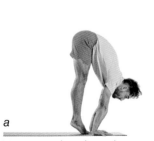
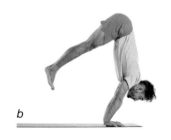
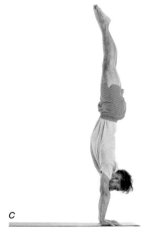

Vinyasa to handstand

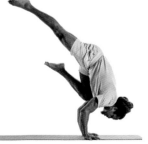
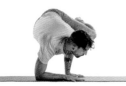
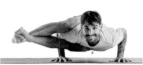

Hurdlers pose to one-leg crow position

Funky arm balance variations to the side inversions

Astavakrasana to koundinyasana

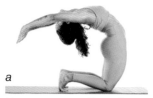 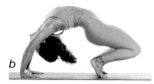 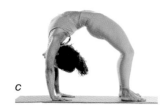

a   b   c

Ustrasana to urdhva dhanurasana

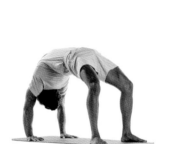 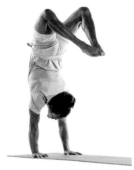 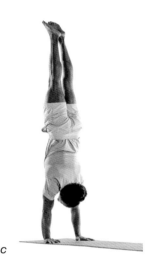

a   b   c

Urdhva dhanurasana to standing or to handstand

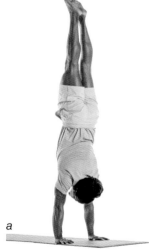 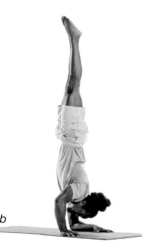 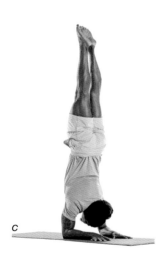

a   b   c

Handstand to forearm stand transition

To learn more creative options in your practice, seek out a certified Rocket vinyasa teacher who can guide you into more playful renditions of the series.

Practicing Drills for Skills

Outside of your practice, there are practical drills that will increase your strength, mobility, and flexibility. While these drills are not yoga per se, they can quickly boost your progress and help to build awareness of your areas of weakness. Practice these drills as homework when you're not in the middle of your practice. These are also fun to do outside in the park. Take your practice off the mat and into the world!

Drills for Improving Handstands

Walking on Hands

It's important to feel comfortable upside down and be willing to catch yourself with your hands if you lose your balance. This is also an exercise that is fun to learn. You do not have to be perfect at handstand walking to take advantage of the skills it will teach you.

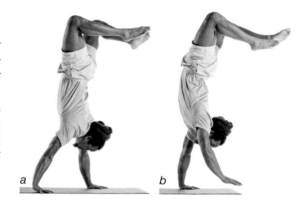

Cartwheels

This is another fun practice that will help with controlled exits from your handstands. Practice cartwheeling on both the right and left sides, slowing the cartwheel to extend the time you spend on your hands. Play with bringing the legs together midcartwheel before stepping out.

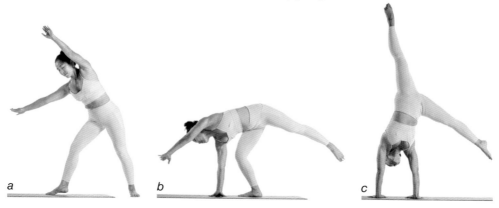

Walking Sideways on a Wall

This can be challenging at first. Do a supported handstand with the wall behind you. Shift your weight to the right hand, and step your left hand toward your right hand. Then, shift your weight to your left hand and walk your right hand out to the right. Keep shifting your weight from hand to hand, stepping each hand out as you move to the side. Once you can take a few steps to the right and left, you will gain more control over maintaining a center and not falling to the side.

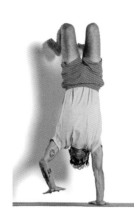

Pike or Tuck

Learn how to access the anterior and posterior tilt of the pelvis while in a handstand. These actions can be small or exaggerated. Any type of exaggeration is considered an advanced technique. Subtle control of this area will produce a stronger balance on the ground. Training both the pike and the tuck techniques will help you to find your balance from the core of the body instead of using your legs to balance you.

You can practice using a wall for support or in the center of the room. While in a handstand, bring the legs to the pike position, moving your legs slightly forward to the front of the body. Simultaneously, allow the sacrum and pelvis to extend to the back of the body as a counterbalance. This is not a straight line. Instead, you will have a slight curve in the lower-lumbar area and softness in the glutes. Keep the shoulders stacked and avoid arching the upper back. Bring the legs back up to a full handstand.

For a tuck, start in a handstand and tighten the glutes and tuck the tailbone with a small push of the pubic bone forward. Let the head drop between the shoulders and shift your gaze behind you.

Explore holding the handstand for longer periods of time (even with a teacher's support) so you can work both the tuck and pike actions together. Your goal is to find the balance between the two actions where you feel most comfortable.

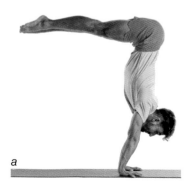

a

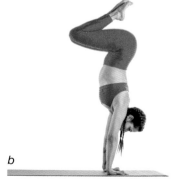

b

(continued)

Drills for Improving Handstands *(continued)*

Straddle Press

This exercise is best done with a partner but can also be done with a wall for support. This will train the muscles needed to support the eventual handstand that you will master on your own. If you're using a wall, come to a full handstand, then rest your hips on the wall. Slowly straddle your legs out to each side, moving with control, and lowering them as far as you can while maintaining control. Bring the legs back up to a full handstand. To do this with a partner, they stand in front of you and hold your hips and support your shoulders as you straddle press up to a handstand.

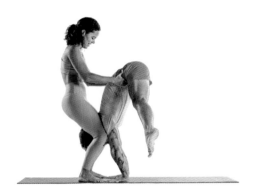

Drills to Improve Seated Vinyasa Technique

• Practice your planks! This will help bring shoulder strength and stability to the shoulder girdle.

• Using blocks under both hands, practice lolasana (page 107). Keep the knees tight to the chest and the feet tucked in. Keeping that contracted body position, allow the body to swing like a pendulum. This will start to bring the motion of the vinyasa into the shoulders.

• From a cross-legged seated position, press both hands into the ground and jump back directly into a chaturanga. Reverse the movement. From a high plank, jump the feet directly into a cross-legged seated position between the hands. The art and practice is in the struggle. Be willing to keep working on it, and wiggle the feet through one at a time. It will get smoother with practice, so don't give up.

• Sock drills on a wooden or tile floor can help to decrease the friction and allow you to slide through the actions. Put on a pair of socks. From a high plank, use your core to pull the legs through the arms to a seated position. Then lift the hips, and push the legs back through the arms to a push-up position. Do 10 to 20 repetitions every day.

Drills for Improving Flexibility

Choose specific postures from the series that challenge you. Practice these alone slowly and with awareness, extending the holds to three to five minutes a pose. Doing this slowly will stretch the body much deeper than the active method used in Rocket vinyasa. Be gentle coming out of the stretch.

Moon Days and Ladies Holidays

Unlike classical ashtanga that observes full moons and new moons with a day of rest, Rocket yoga asks that you listen to your body and your own needs to determine whether you should practice. If you are feeling mentally and physically great, there is no reason why you shouldn't practice.

Similarly, Rocket yoga does not subscribe to the traditional notion for women to refrain from practice while on their menstrual cycle. Little medical evidence supports this reasoning and echoes a time when women were seen as dirty during their cycle and were not allowed to be in a temple or shala. Women, you are asked to listen to your body and practice if it feels right to do so or take time off if the body feels a need to rest. Rocket yoga empowers each student to determine for themselves what to practice, how to practice, and how often to practice.

Practicing Yoga During Pregnancy

The room for creativity and modification makes Rocket sequences perfect for the body as it changes during the phases of pregnancy. Pregnancy makes mothers strong. It's beneficial to support this strength that will be used for the birthing process. Consult with your primary care physician before beginning this physical training just as you would before starting any other physical practice. It would be ideal to have an existing practice in Rocket vinyasa and then make the changes for this new adventure. It is not recommended to begin a Rocket practice for the first time during pregnancy. Instead, find a certified prenatal teacher who can guide you into the practice with more support.

These are some of the general principles to keep in mind if you're practicing Rocket yoga during pregnancy.

- Allow the practice to change and shift during the stages of the pregnancy.
- Listen to your body and do only what feels appropriate.
- Remember that when pregnant, you have 40 to 60 percent more blood in your body, and therefore, your heart is working much faster than normal. You can feel out of breath and tired more easily.
- The relaxin hormone is secreted into the body at conception and stays in the body for several months after delivery. The hormone is responsible for helping to soften the connective tissues in preparation for childbirth, so be careful not to overstretch during this time, even if it feels good. Stay within the boundaries set in your body before pregnancy.

- Pregnancy produces a naturally low blood sugar state. Although classical ashtanga and Rocket yoga are traditionally practiced on an empty stomach, pregnant women should eat or drink juice before class—even if it is just a small snack.

Here are some specific things to be aware of while practicing:

- You want to create space in your abdominal region for the growing baby. Engaging the abdominal muscles constricts this region and should not be practiced. This means not applying uddiyana bandha. Focus instead on engaging the mula bandha and strengthening the pelvic floor.
- Inversions during pregnancy are contraindicated. Instead of shoulder stands and headstands, a safe alternative is legs up the wall. This is partially because of blood flow, but it is also because of the danger of falling. Increased blood volume along with pressure on the umbilical cord when inverted can create complications that put you at risk. If you already have a strong, stable inversion practice, you may feel confident practicing inversions for short periods.
- Lying on your back or on your right side can constrict the blood flow and the flow of blood to the uterus. If you do lie on the floor, lie on your left side. If you want to lie on your back, use bolsters to support your back so you stay on an incline.
- Deep spinal twists can create stress for the already overstretched ligaments in the pelvic region. Twists are appropriate, but they should be done lightly, ideally not crossing the midline of the body. In seated or standing twists, avoid twisting into a position that compresses the abdomen, instead twisting away from the compression of the belly.
- Sometimes in class you may simply not feel like practicing or may not be capable of practicing certain postures. Here are options for when a class is doing postures that are not appropriate for your body:
  - *Viparita karani*: Legs up the wall is a great inversion that alleviates swelling in the ankles by taking the pressure off the feet and reversing the flow of blood.
  - *Child's pose*: Keep the knees wide apart, making ample room for the belly between the thighs.
  - *Squats at the wall*: Keep the back against the wall with the toes wider than the heels. Slowly move down the wall into a squat.
  - *Squats away from the wall*: Stand with the legs wide apart and the toes turned out. Keep the upper body straight as you slowly lower your hips into a squat. You can place a block under the seat or you can hold the squat with your own strength.

Rocket yoga is about self-expression and freedom of movement. It is a celebration of movement through the discipline of yoga. Any modifications taken to invite more ease and freedom into the practice, to challenge the mind, or to discover the limits of the body are absolutely encouraged.

REFERENCES

Crooks, D. 2017. "Larry Schultz." *Yogi Times*, December 14, 2017. www.yogitimes.com/review/larry-schultz-yoga-teachers-san-francisco.

Cushman, A. 1995. "Power Yoga." *Yoga Journal*, Jan/Feb.

Lurrey, D. 2021. "The Rocket, a Tribute to Larry Schultz." *Ekhart Yoga*, January 27, 2021. www.ekhartyoga.com/articles/practice/the-rocket-a-tribute-to-larry-schultz.

Russel, M. 2018. "Meet Our Founder." It's Yoga International, May 14, 2018. https://itsyoga.com/meet-our-founder.

ABOUT THE AUTHOR

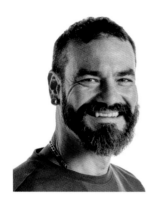

David Kyle, RYT-500, CMT-1000, is the founder of Progressive Ashtanga Vinyasa Yoga School and is the director of all progressive ashtanga teacher trainings and intensives. He was a dedicated student of Larry Schultz, private yoga instructor for the Grateful Dead and the creator of Rocket yoga. Kyle is the highest-trained student of Larry Schultz in both primary series modifications and the Rocket series, and he is the sole owner and operator of trainings and international relations in Rocket®.

With over 20 years of yoga experience and over 30 years in body movement and the healing arts, Kyle has offered advanced yoga trainings worldwide, including the United States, Canada, South America, Mexico, China, and Europe. Rooted in the traditional ashtanga method, he makes use of the fundamental strengths of the practice while allowing for students and teachers to find empowerment in their practice through creativity, endurance, and rhythm.

ABOUT THE PROJECT EDITOR

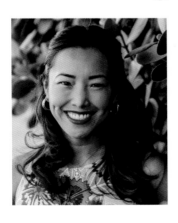

Christine Fenerty is a nutrition coach and yoga teacher, a culinary school graduate, and a student of ashtanga. Between baking and sun salutations, she sparks others to follow their purpose through wellness coaching, international retreats, and helping others to bring their projects to fruition. She lives in Port Saint Lucie, Florida. You can find her at www.christinefenerty.com.

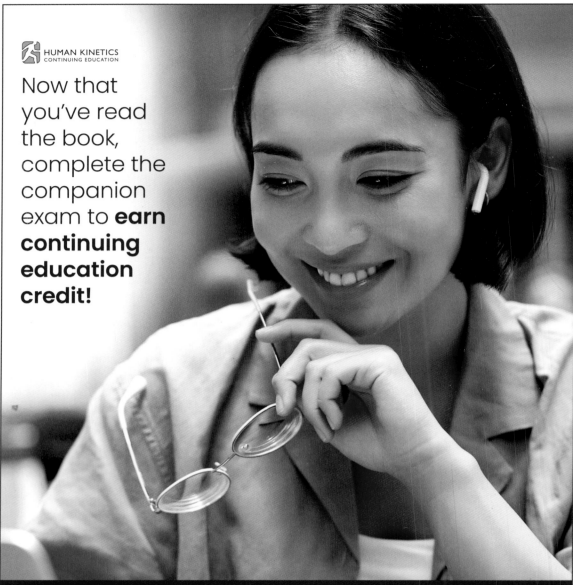
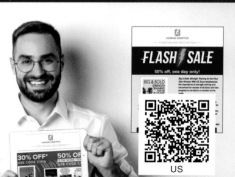